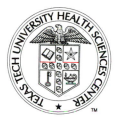

# An Atlas of Planar and SPECT Bone Scans

# An Atlas of Planar and SPECT Bone Scans

**Ignac Fogelman,** BSc, MD, FRCP
Director of Nuclear Medicine, Guy's Hospital, London

**B David Collier,** MD
Associate Professor of Radiology and Orthopaedic Surgery
Director of Nuclear Medicine, Medical College of Wisconsin

**Martin Dunitz**
London

**The C.V. Mosby Company**
St. Louis ● Washington, D.C. ● Toronto

1989

First published in the United Kingdom in 1989
by Martin Dunitz Ltd, 154 Camden High Street, London NW1 0NE

Distributed in the United States, Mexico, Central America, and South America by
The C.V. Mosby Company,
11830 Westline Industrial Drive, St. Louis, Missouri 63146, U.S.A.

Distributed in Canada by The C.V. Mosby Company, Ltd., 5420 Finch Avenue East,
Scarborough, Ontario, Canada M1S 4P2

**Library of Congress Cataloging-in-Publication Data**

Fogelman, Ignac, 1948–
    An atlas of planar and SPECT bone scans.

    Includes index.
    1. Bones–Diseases–Diagnosis–Atlases.
2. Bones–Radionuclide imaging–Atlases.
I. Collier, David. II. Title. [DNLM: 1. Bone and
Bones–radionuclide imaging–atlases. 2. Tomography,
Emission Computed–methods–atlases. WE 17 F6555a]
RC930.5.F64   1988        617'.3707575        88–13551
ISBN 0-8016-3296-X

Laserset by Scribe Design, Gillingham, Kent
Origination by Adroit Photolitho Ltd, Birmingham
Printed and bound in England by Cambridge University Press

*This book is dedicated to Coral, Jan and our children*

# Preface

Bone scanning is an important diagnostic technique, which can profitably be applied to almost all aspects of skeletal pathology, and this atlas will prove to be an invaluable aid to those whose work centres around the investigation of the skeleton. The over 900 illustrations represent the work of two busy hospital departments, both with large patient populations but, nevertheless, with often quite different clinical practices.

The book has been carefully structured to facilitate problem solving. We have also distilled our own experience into compact and accessible 'Teaching points', which are found extensively throughout the text.

By combining his knowledge of nuclear medicine with the case material and analyses presented in this atlas, the practitioner should be able to make optimal interpretations of planar and SPECT bone scan images. As particular emphasis has been placed on clinical application, those working in specialties such as orthopaedics, oncology, rheumatology and endocrinology will find much of interest and direct practical relevance.

# Acknowledgments

It would have been impossible to produce a nuclear medicine atlas of planar and SPECT bone scans without the assistance of our colleagues and support, if not sympathy, from our families.

While many individuals have played a role in the creation of this atlas the contributions of several are particularly notable.

At Guy's Hospital we are grateful to Katie Pert, who photographed many of the illustrations, and to the audio-visual services for producing the prints, as well as Carolyn Bishop and Marion Blagg for typing the manuscript.

At the Medical College of Wisconsin we are grateful to Drs Arthur Z Krasnow and Guillermo F Carrera for their assistance in organizing the material.

We acknowledge the skill and hard work of our technical staff, who ensured consistent high-quality work.

In addition we wish to thank the following doctors who provided material and without whose contributions this atlas would be incomplete:

Drs M D Francis, M Hutchinson, A Schoutens, L Smith, H Wahner, P Wraight, A Z Krasnow, P Veluvolu, J R Sty, S Arnold, R P Johnson, R S Hellman, A T Isitman, H S Kohn, G N Guten and P Donahue.

We are indebted to Professor Michael Maisey for his encouragement throughout this project.

Finally, we would like to express our thanks to the staff of Martin Dunitz for their patient co-operation.

**I FOGELMAN**
**B D COLLIER**
London 1988

# Contents

# List of SPECT images

# Introduction 1

The bone scan is the most frequently performed nuclear medicine imaging procedure. In current clinical practice, it is often used as a high sensitivity screening test, which in most clinical situations outperforms conventional X-ray for the detection of skeletal pathology. At other times, the bone scan is valuable as a functional test of bone metabolism that complements the anatomical detail available from conventional X-ray, computed tomography (CT) or magnetic resonance imaging (MRI).

The continuous growth in bone scanning since the introduction of technetium-99m ($^{99m}$Tc) labelled tracers more than 10 years ago has progressed alongside improvements in imaging techniques. Each new generation of gamma cameras has provided the nuclear medicine practitioner with improved bone scan images. The recent introduction of single photon emission computed tomography (SPECT) enhances the bone scan by providing cross-sectional anatomical detail and image contrast that previously was unavailable. Equally important to the recent growth in bone scanning have been the newer clinical applications, not only in oncology but also in orthopaedics, sports medicine and rheumatology.

This atlas considers in detail adult bone scanning with $^{99m}$Tc-labelled diphosphonates, and includes a limited selection of paediatric bone scans as well. The mechanisms of tracer uptake and techniques for both planar and SPECT bone scanning are first described. This chapter is followed by a carefully structured presentation of normal bone scans, normal variants, artefacts and pitfalls, frequently encountered scan 'patterns', an extensive collection of scans showing bone abnormalities due to a wide variety of malignant and benign skeletal pathology, and miscellaneous extraskeletal bone scan findings. Other nuclear medicine techniques, such as gallium-67 scanning, and other imaging modalities, for example, conventional X-ray, CT and MRI are considered in passing only as they relate to the bone scan cases presented.

## Mechanisms of tracer uptake

Bone scanning is almost exclusively performed using $^{99m}$Tc-labelled diphosphonate (Figure 1.1) which shows exquisite sensitivity for skeletal abnormality. The technique has the limitation that scan appearances may be non-specific; however, in many clinical situations recognizable patterns of scan abnormality are seen which often suggest a specific diagnosis.

The mechanism of tracer uptake on to bone is not fully understood but it is believed that diphosphonate is adsorbed on to the surface of bone, with particular affinity for sites of new bone formation (Figures 1.2, 1.3). It is thought that diphosphonate uptake on bone primarily reflects osteoblastic activity but is also dependent on skeletal vascularity. Thus bone scan images provide a functional display of skeletal activity. As functional change in bone occurs earlier than gross structural change, the bone scan will often detect abnormalities before they are seen on an X-ray. Any diphosphonate which is not taken up by bone is excreted via the urinary tract, and in a normal study the kidneys are clearly visualized on the bone scan; indeed there are many examples of renal pathology which have been detected for the first time on the bone scan.

It is also recognized that, on occasion, there may be uptake of $^{99m}$Tc diphosphonate at non-skeletal sites. There have been many situations reported where this can occur, but it is believed that in all cases the common factor is the presence of local microcalcification.

# Chemical structure of diphosphonates

**Figure 1.1**

Chemical structure of diphosphonate compounds used for bone scanning. At the present time MDP is the most widely used agent. HEDP, hydroxyethylidene diphosphonate; MDP, methylene diphosphonate; HMDP, hydroxymethylene diphosphonate; DPD, dicarboxypropane diphosphonate.

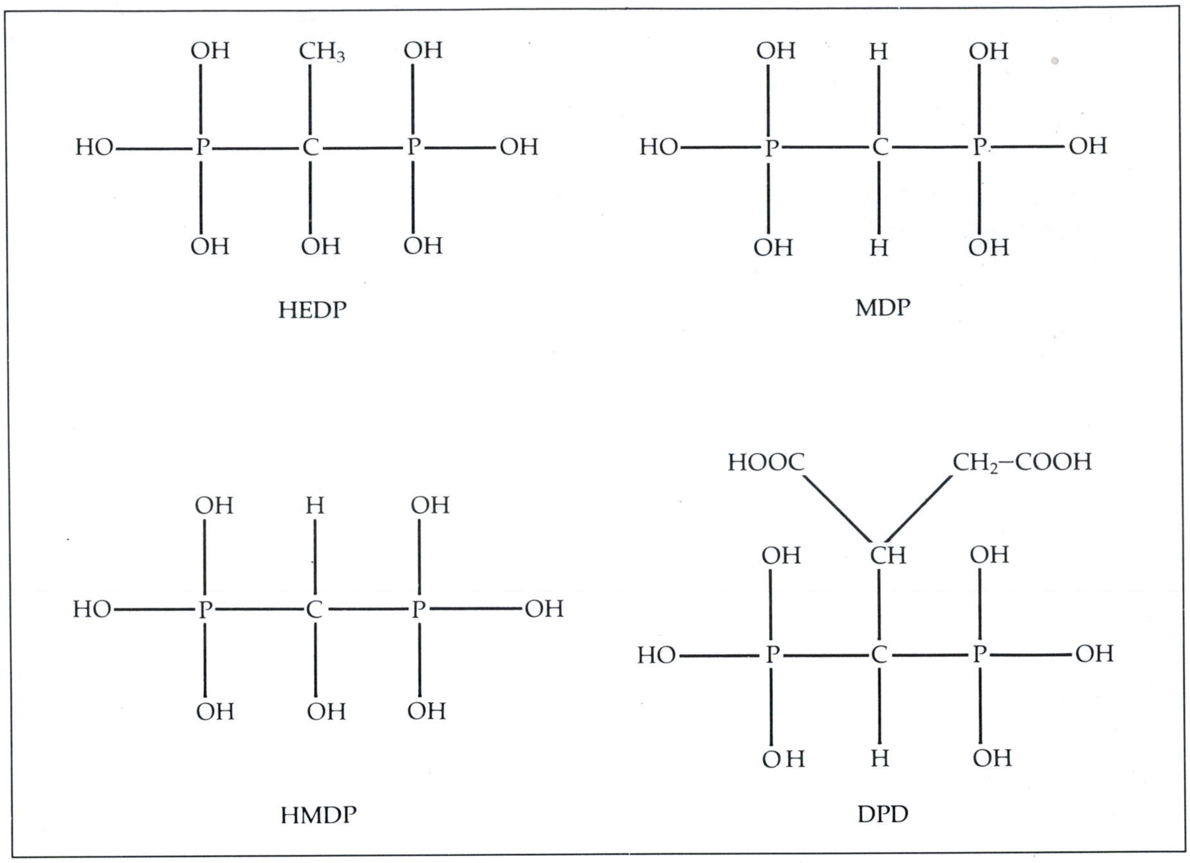

# Mechanism of diphosphonate uptake on bone

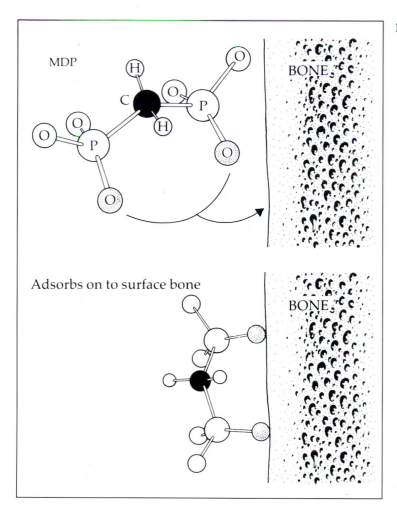

**Figure 1.2**

MDP

Adsorbs on to surface bone

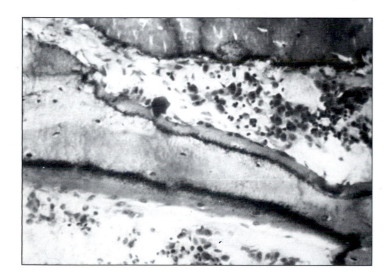

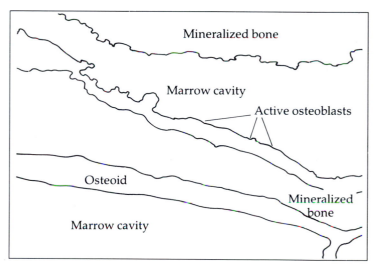

Mineralized bone

Marrow cavity

Active osteoblasts

Osteoid

Mineralized bone

Marrow cavity

**Figure 1.3**

Microautoradiograph of rabbit bone showing adsorption of ³H–HEDP on bone surfaces. The heavy concentration of silver grains is at the interface between osteoid and bone, ie, at the site where mineralization occurs.

# Bone scan techniques

A brief outline of the author's protocols for both planar and SPECT bone scanning is given in Tables 1.1–1.5. When compared with planar imaging, SPECT offers both cross-sectional anatomical detail and improved image contrast. SPECT removes from each diagnostic image the activity originating outside the tomographic plane of medical interest. For example, in the hip the acetabulum extends around and behind the femoral head. Therefore, a planar bone scan abnormality within the femoral head may be obscured by activity originating in the underlying acetabulum. Using SPECT it is possible to separate underlying and overlying distributions of activity into sequential tomographic planes. For this reason, SPECT often improves detection of an abnormality within the femoral head itself.

The improvement in image contrast and anatomical detail available with SPECT must be weighed against the superior spatial resolution of planar bone scanning. For the high resolution bone SPECT technique used at the authors' institutions, spatial resolution for the spine is no better than 14 mm full width half maximum. This is compared with 8 mm or better resolution (at a depth of 5 cm or less using a high resolution collimator) for a state-of-the-art planar bone scan. When evaluating the hands, feet or other relatively small and superficial bony structures, high resolution planar bone scanning usually provides superior images. However, SPECT can make a valuable contribution to the examination of large, anatomically complex structures such as the spine, hips and knees. SPECT may also be essential for examining small bony structures which one may want to image individually. For example, SPECT can isolate the temporomandibular joint (TMJ) from activity originating in other bony structures of the face and base of the skull.

SPECT supplements but does not replace planar bone scanning. Therefore, the time and expense of SPECT is an addition to the bone scan examination. Since many patients complaining of bone pain may benefit from a dynamic study and blood pool image, SPECT often becomes the fourth component of a patient's bone scan. At our institutions, the imaging sequence for patients without a history or suspicion of malignancy who complain of back, hip, knee or TMJ pain is as follows:

1 Dynamic study (2–5 seconds per frame)
2 Blood pool image (500000 counts)
3 Planar bone scan
4 SPECT bone scan

Patients referred to nuclear medicine for the evaluation of osteomyelitis, orthopaedic disorders or sports injuries require bone scans that are carefully tailored to their individual needs. For example, osteomyelitis should be evaluated with a dynamic study, blood pool image and subsequent delayed planar bone scan images. The evaluation of orthopaedic disorders and sports injuries usually calls for planar bone scans which show the best possible anatomical detail. This requires high resolution collimation and may call for special positioning, such as oblique views of the shoulder or plantar views of the feet. Even when optimal high resolution planar bone scans have been obtained, the addition of SPECT to these orthopaedic examinations will frequently yield further valuable diagnostic information.

When evaluating oncology patients, the authors prefer to obtain multiple overlapping bone scan images rather than use whole body imaging techniques. Multiple overlapping 'spot' images always have higher resolution than the total body images obtained with a scanning mechanism. The superior resolution of 'spot' images aids detection of bone metastases and facilitates accurate anatomical localization of skeletal lesions.

## Table 1.1 Protocols for planar bone scanning

*Patient preparation*
Encourage fluids and frequent voiding
Remove metal objects and ask patient to void
    before scan

*Adult dose*
550 MBq $^{99m}$Tc-MDP

*Scanning 3–4 hours after injection*
1  Whole body technique; or
2  Multiple overlapping bone scan views
   ■ Low energy all-purpose, or low energy high
        resolution collimator
   ■ 500 000 to 1 000 000 count thoracic spine scan
   ■ Obtain all other scans for same length of time

## Table 1.2 Planar bone scanning pitfalls

| Pitfall | Result |
| --- | --- |
| Over 5 cm collimator-to-patient separation | Loss resolution |
| Wrong energy windows | Loss resolution |
| Low count study | 'Grainy' scan |
| $^{99m}$Tc-MDP impurities | Increased background activity and soft tissue uptake |
| Renal failure | Increased background activity |
| Slight patient motion | Loss resolution |
| Obesity | Increased background and scattered activity |

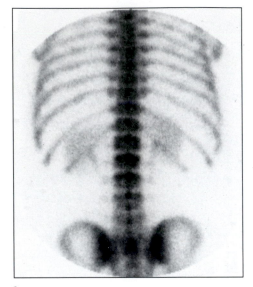
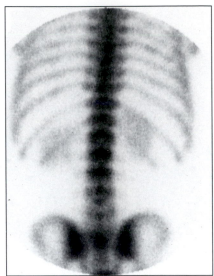
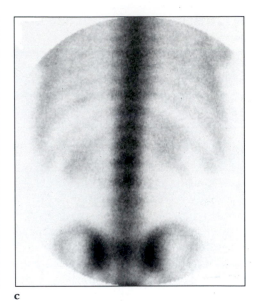

a         b         c

**Figure 1.4**

Posterior view bone scans of the thoracolumbar spine obtained with the collimator **(a)** in close apposition to the patient's back, **(b)** 13 cm from the back and **(c)** 25 cm from the back. It is apparent that as the collimator is moved away from the patient, spatial resolution decreases and image clarity deteriorates.

## Table 1.3 Protocols for SPECT bone scanning

*Adult dose*
925 MBq $^{99m}$Tc-MDP

*Acquisition 3–4 hours later*
64 × 64 matrix (400 mm field-of-view gamma camera)

*General method*
Low energy all-purpose collimator
20 seconds per projection, 64 projections over 360 degrees

*High resolution method (option for lumbar spine)*
High resolution collimator
25 seconds per projection, 64 projections over 360 degrees

*Processing*
Uniformity correction
Hanning filter (frequency cut-off = 0.8 cycle/cm pre-processing)
Reconstruction by filtered back–projection with Ramp filter
No attenuation correction
6 mm (one pixel) thick transaxial, sagittal and coronal images

*Display*
Use linear grey scale map for TMJ, lumbar spine and knee SPECT
Use log grey scale when searching for femoral head avascular necrosis

## Table 1.4 Special patient positioning for SPECT bone scanning

| Bony structure | Special positioning | Comments |
|---|---|---|
| Knees | 5–7.5 cm pad between knees; secure knees with straps to prevent motion<br>Secure feet in neutral position to prevent rotation | For obese patients both knees may not fit in field of view |
| Hips and pelvis | Empty bladder before examination<br>Position hips symmetrically and secure knees and/or feet to prevent motion | Bladder filling during examination creates artefacts |
| Lumbar spine | Keep arms out of field of view<br>A pillow under the knees may relieve back pain | Patients with back pain often move during the examination |
| TMJ | Secure neck in comfortable hyperextension<br>Instruct patient not to talk | Check lateral view to be sure the chin is in the field of view |

## Table 1.5 Gamma camera quality control for planar and SPECT bone scanning

*Daily*

Extrinsic flood for uniformity check:

- 3.0 million counts, 400 mm field-of-view camera
- 4.5 million counts, 500 mm field-of-view camera

*Weekly*

Update energy correction per manufacturer recommendation

Intrinsic flood for uniformity check:

- 3.0 million counts, 400 mm field-of-view camera
- 4.5 million counts, 500 mm field-of-view camera

Update tomographic centre of rotation

Update high count extrinsic flood for uniformity correction:

- 30 million counts for $64 \times 64$ matrix
- 120 million counts for $128 \times 128$ matrix

*Monthly*

Image bar phantom for check of planar resolution
Image tomographic phantom (optional)

# Pattern recognition

## 2

In order to be able to recognize an abnormal bone scan, the physician must be familiar with normal bone scan appearances and the commonly seen variants. While the scan appearances may be non-specific, recognizable patterns of abnormality are often seen which may suggest a specific diagnosis. An experienced observer will regularly be correct in suggesting that a specific diagnosis has a high probability of being present. However, even an expert will be mistaken from time to time. A bone scan should not be considered to be a definitive investigation, but rather one that provides high sensitivity for lesion detection which often will require further investigation.

The following patterns of scan findings will be considered:

- Normal bone scan
- Variants
- Artefacts and pitfalls
- Metastases
- Marrow hyperplasia
- Trauma
- Arthritis
- Metabolic bone disease
- Vertebral collapse
- Paget's disease.

# Normal bone scan

■ Departments vary in their policy as to whether to obtain a whole body bone scan, or multiple overlapping images of the skeleton. In most cases the bone scan is requested because of its high sensitivity for detecting skeletal metastases. The present authors believe that it is important to obtain images with the highest possible resolution and therefore favour obtaining overlapping views. Any scanning gamma camera producing a single image of the whole skeleton has lower resolution than the same camera used in the static mode. The main reason for this is that resolution falls rapidly as the distance between the collimator face and the patient increases. Therefore, 'spot' views will always show higher resolution than those obtained with a scanning mechanism.

**Figure 2.1**

An example of a normal bone scan: **(a)** anterior and **(b)** posterior views. Note that there is clear visualization of the whole skeleton. The count rate is highest in those parts of the skeleton which are metabolically most active. These areas generally contain a high percentage of trabecular bone and are subject to considerable stress, eg, the axial skeleton. The most important feature in a normal bone scan is symmetry about the mid-line in the sagittal plane. The left and right halves of the body should be virtually mirror images of each other. There should be uniform uptake of tracer throughout most of the skeleton, but some exceptions do arise, as will be discussed in the variants section (see pages 30–37). Note that the kidneys are clearly visualized on a normal bone scan because the diphosphonate which is not taken up by the skeleton is excreted via the urinary tract.

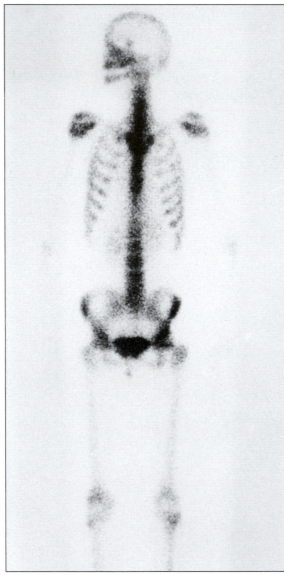

a

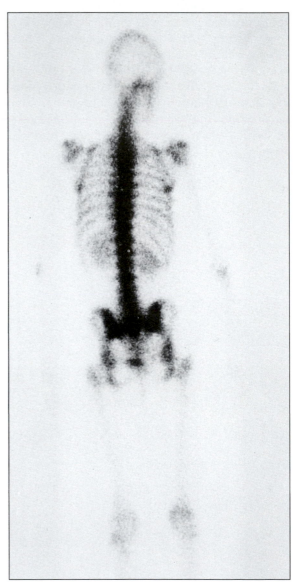

b

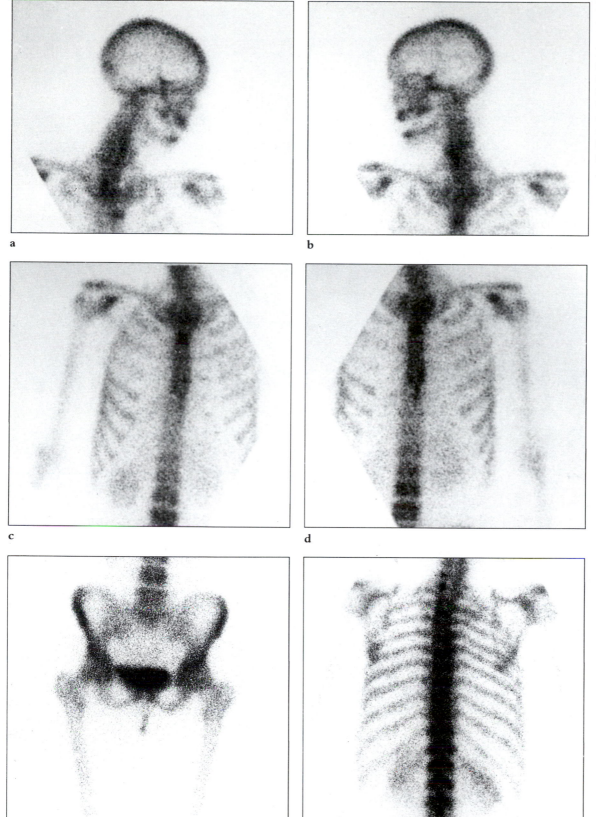

a

b

c

d

e

f

**Figure 2.2**

Normal bone scan views: **(a)** right lateral skull, **(b)** left lateral skull, **(c)** right anterior thorax, **(d)** left anterior thorax, **(e)** anterior pelvis, **(f)** posterior thoracic spine, **(g)** posterior lumbar spine/pelvis, **(h)** femora, **(i)** tibiae, **(j)** feet, and **(k)** lower forearms and hands.

**Figure 2.2** *continued*

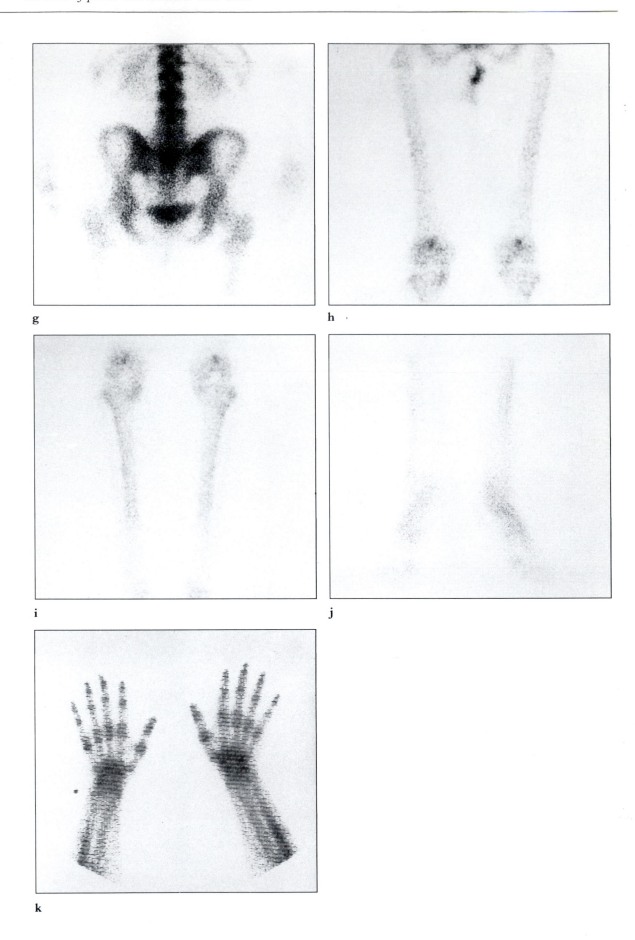

g

h

i

j

k

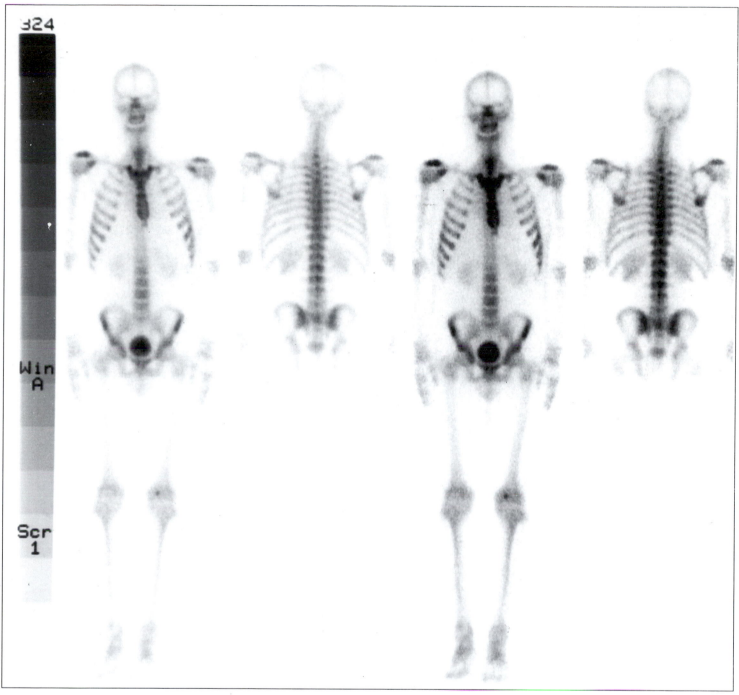

a

**Figure 2.3**

An essentially normal bone scan in a 26-year-old male volunteer. Total body images **(a)** along with 'spot' views, obtained using a high resolution collimator, of the **(b, c)** skull, **(d, e)** spine, anterior **(f)** and posterior **(g)** pelvis, **(h)** anterior chest, **(i)** anterior right arm, **(j)** anterior left arm, **(k)** hands, **(l)** femora, anterior **(m)** and right lateral **(n)** knees, and **(o)** feet. While this is an essentially normal study it should be noted that increased tracer uptake is seen in the left patella and the right 5th PIP joint. The volunteer was symp- tom free and had no history of arthritis or trauma at these sites. These bone scans were photographed using a digital display which allows the operator to choose the appropriate intensity and contrast.

**Figure 2.3** *continued*

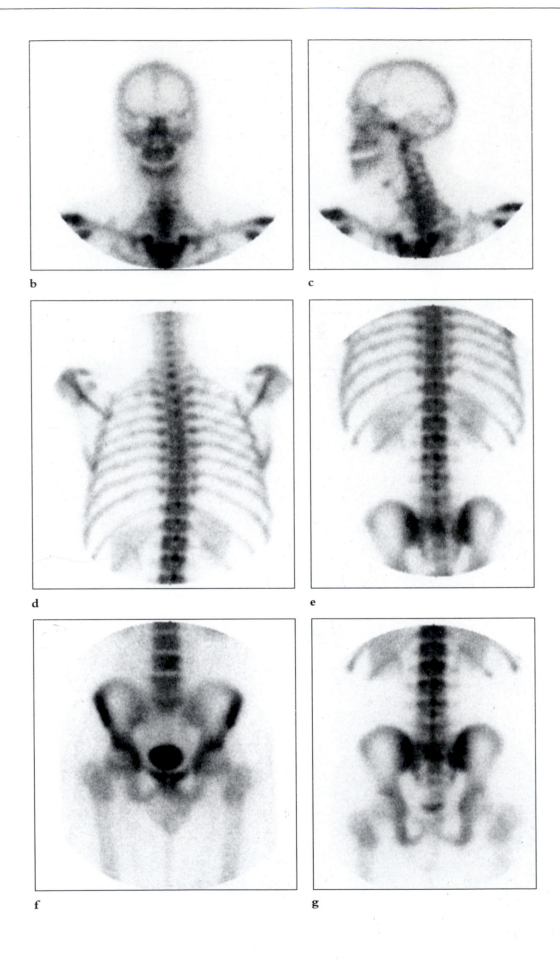

b

c

d

e

f

g

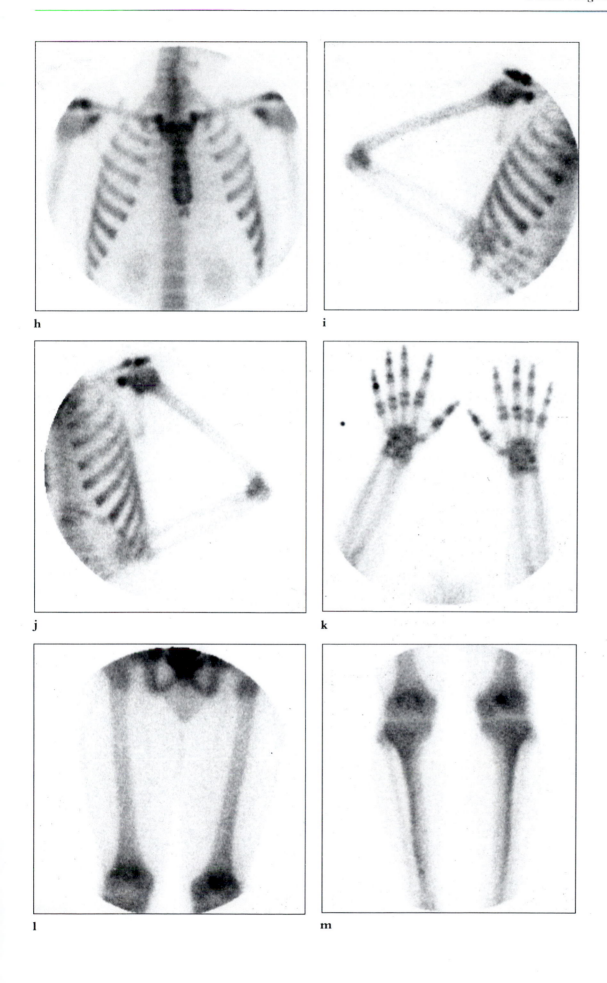

h

i

j

k

l

m

**Figure 2.3** *continued*

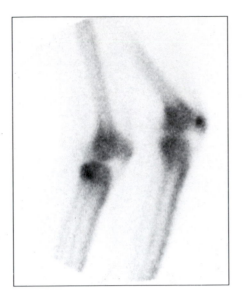

n

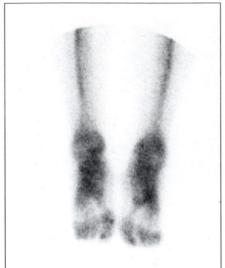

o

---

## ■ Teaching point

---

■
When examining young adults in whom there is no history of malignancy, arthritis or trauma, slight increased tracer uptake occasionally is seen at asymptomatic juxta-articular sites in the hands, feet and knees. In the authors' experience, no patient with this combination of clinical and scintigraphic findings has had significant skeletal pathology. While careful correlation with history and clinical data is important, X-ray correlation usually is unwarranted.

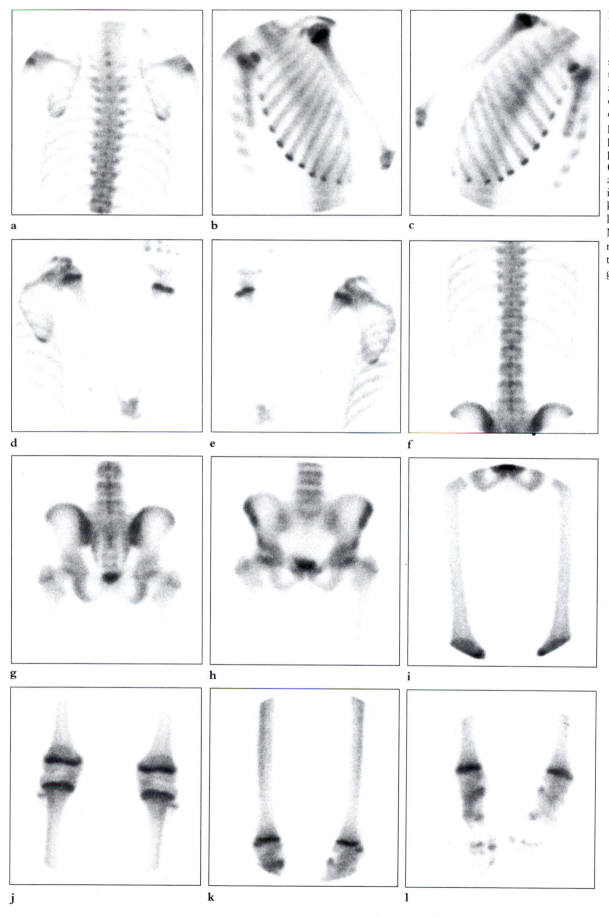

**Figure 2.4**

Normal bone scan of a 16-year-old boy. Bone scan views: **(a)** posterior thoracic spine, **(b)** left anterior oblique (LAO) chest, **(c)** right anterior oblique (RAO) chest, **(d)** posterior right arm, **(e)** posterior left arm, **(f)** posterior lumbar spine, **(g)** posterior pelvis, **(h)** anterior pelvis, **(i)** anterior femora, **(j)** anterior knees, **(k)** anterior lower legs and **(l)** anterior feet. Note the prominent yet normal tracer uptake at the metabolically active growth plates.

**Figure 2.5**

Normal bone scan of a 3-year-old boy. Bone scan views: **(a)** right lateral skull, **(b)** left lateral skull, **(c)** posterior thoracic spine, **(d)** LAO chest, **(e)** RAO chest, **(f)** posterior right arm, **(g)** posterior left arm, **(h)** posterior lumbosacral spine, **(i)** anterior pelvis, **(j)** anterior knees and **(k)** anterior feet. Tracer uptake at the growth plates is particularly prominent at this age.

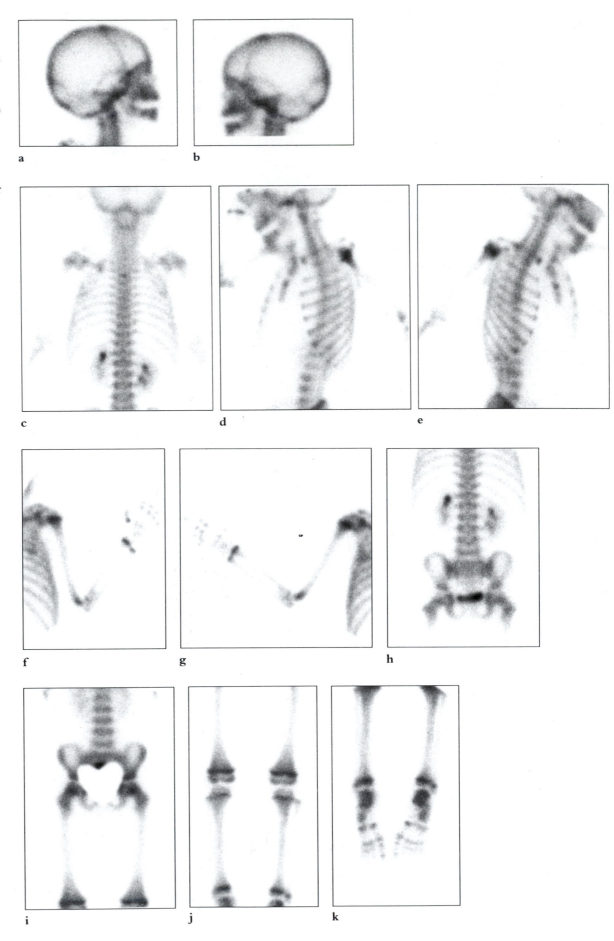

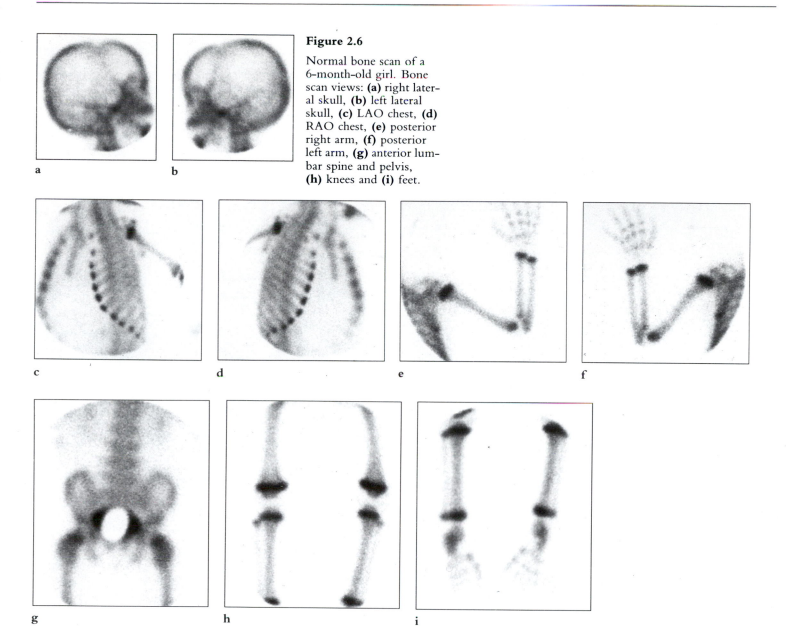

**Figure 2.6**

Normal bone scan of a 6-month-old girl. Bone scan views: **(a)** right lateral skull, **(b)** left lateral skull, **(c)** LAO chest, **(d)** RAO chest, **(e)** posterior right arm, **(f)** posterior left arm, **(g)** anterior lumbar spine and pelvis, **(h)** knees and **(i)** feet.

# 'Three-phrase' bone scan

■ The timing of bone scan images may depend upon the clinical problem under investigation. There is, at present, no complete agreement as to the optimum time interval between injection and static imaging, but it is customary to obtain images at between 2 and 4 hours. In certain circumstances a 'three-phase' bone scan will provide valuable additional information with regard to the vascularity of a lesion. This involves a dynamic flow study of the area of interest, with rapid sequential images taken every 2–5 seconds for 30 seconds. This is followed by a blood pool image at 5 minutes, when the radiopharmaceutical is still predominantly within the vascular compartment. Delayed static images are then obtained at the normal time.

**Figure 2.7**

Normal three-phase bone scan of the lower limbs. Bone scan views: **(a)** dynamic, **(b)** blood pool and **(c)** delayed.

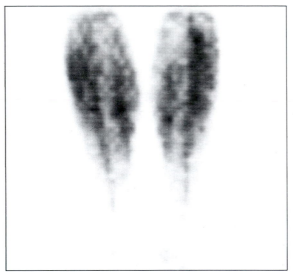

a

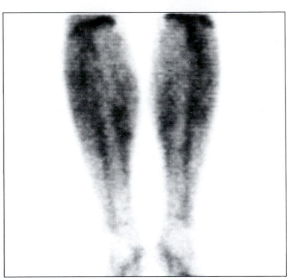

b

c

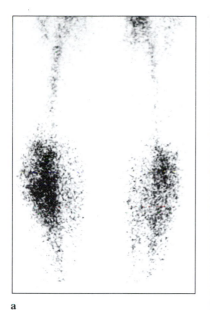
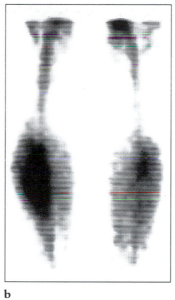
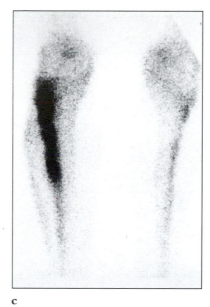

a                    b                    c

**Figure 2.8**

A 17-year-old boy with Ewing's tumour. Three-phase bone scan views: (a) dynamic, (b) blood pool and (c) delayed. There is a massively increased blood flow to the right fibula and associated soft tissue. Delayed images show intense metabolic activity at the upper two-thirds of the right fibula.

# Importance of symmetry

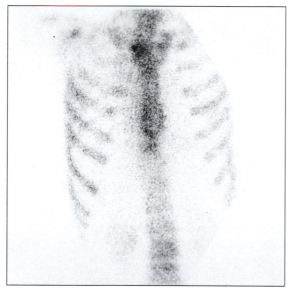
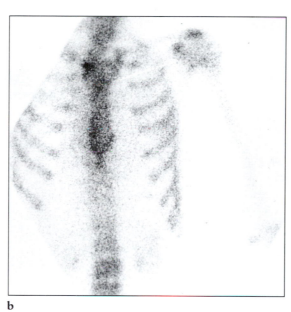

a                                    b

**Figure 2.9**

Bone scan views: (a) right anterior chest, (b) left anterior chest and (c) posterior thoracic spine. This patient has had amputation of the right arm. While this appears obvious, it is easy to over-look such a gross abnormality. In this case there is also increased uptake in the right sternoclavicular joint, reflecting degenerative change.

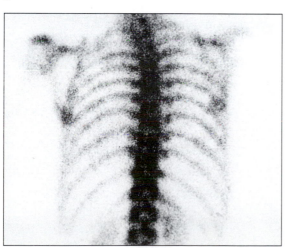

c

## SPECT: single photon emission computed tomography

**Figure 2.10**

Normal SPECT bone scan images of the knee of a 20-year-old man: **(a)** transaxial plane through femoral condyles near the joint line, **(b)** coronal plane through femoral condyles and tibial plateau, and **(c)** sagittal plane through the mid-patella. Note that activity originating in subchondral bone over the medial and lateral compartments is substantially less intense than the activity over the growth plates. Further-more, activity in the patella has an intensity similar to that of the sub-chondral bone in the me-dial and lateral compart-ments. Intensity equal to or greater than the growth plates would indicate the presence of abnormal activity in the patella or bone adjacent to the weight-bearing surfaces.

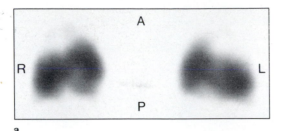

a

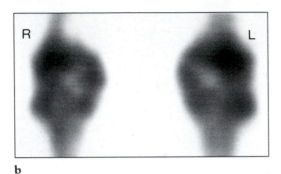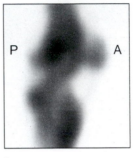

b                                              c

**Figure 2.11**

Anterior view of the right knee.

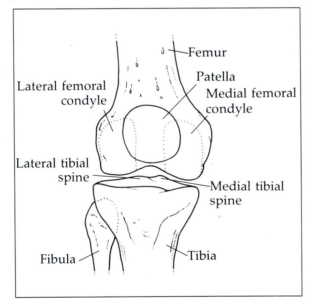

## ■ Teaching point

■ Prominent tracer uptake in the growth plates of long bones may per-sist beyond adolesence and is occa-sionally seen in normal knees of 25–30-year-old patients. The rich vascularity of bone normally present in recently fused growth plates may account for this prominent tracer uptake.

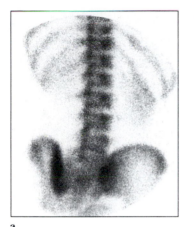

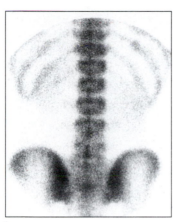

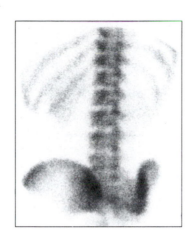

a

b

c

**Figure 2.12**

A normal lumbar spine planar and SPECT bone scan of a 40-year-old man obtained using a high resolution collimator. Planar bone scan views: **(a)** right posterior oblique (RPO), **(b)** posterior, and **(c)** left posterior oblique (LPO). SPECT (8 mm thick) bone scan images: **(d, e)** transaxial (images read from cephalad to caudad), **(f)** coronal (front to back) and **(g)** sagittal (right to left). With SPECT images one can visualize the individual lumbar vertebral bodies, spinal canal, pedicles and spinous processes. This is not possible on planar bone scans, even with high resolution collimation and additional posterior oblique views, as there is superimposed activity originating in the various bony structures of the lumbar spine.

d

**Figure 2.12** *continued*

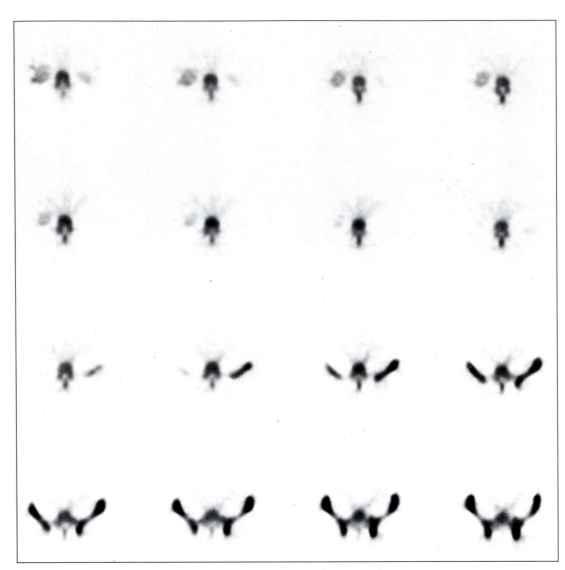

e

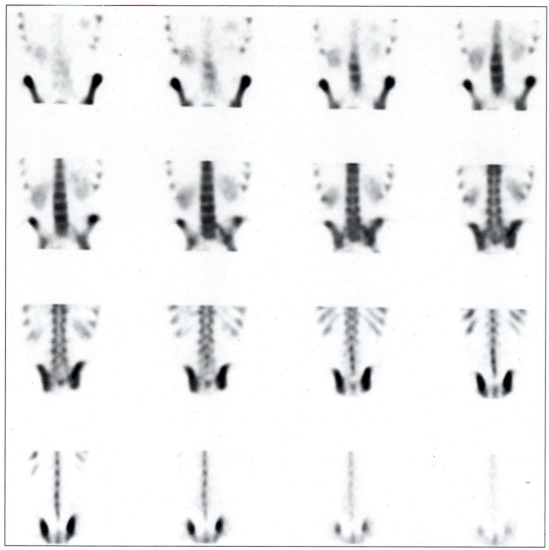

f

**Figure 2.12** *continued*

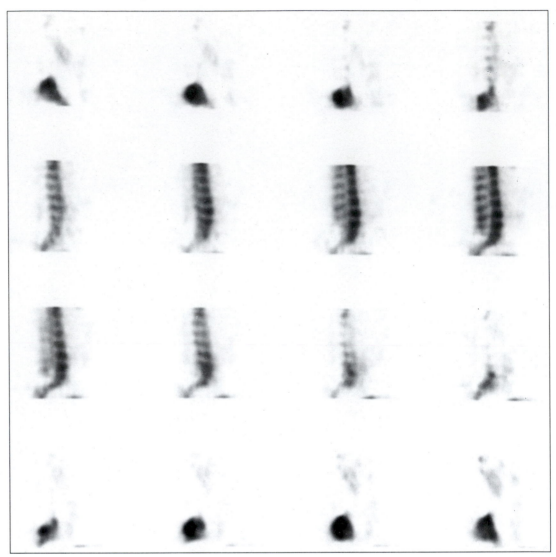

g

## ■ Teaching point

■

When viewing transaxial and coronal
SPECT images, note that the patient's
right side is on the reader's left side.

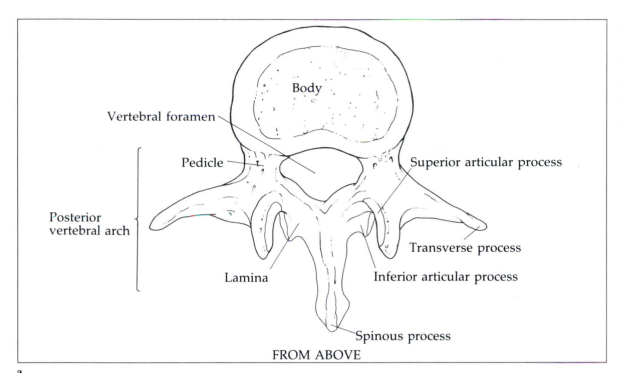

FROM ABOVE

a

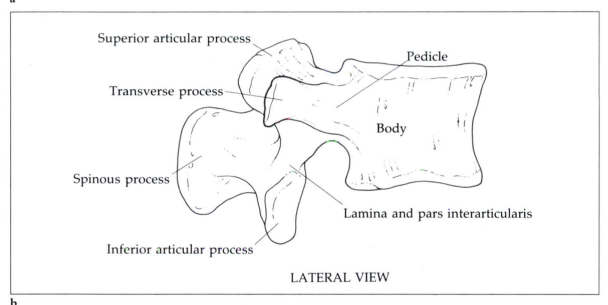

LATERAL VIEW

b

**Figure 2.13**

Second lumbar vertebra **(a)** from above and **(b)** from the lateral side. Note that the parts of the posterior vertebral arch such as the spinous process are resolved on the SPECT bone scans shown in Figure 2.10.

# ■ Teaching points

■ A SPECT bone scan evaluation of the lumbar spine is not complete until the nuclear medicine physician has reviewed all the coronal, sagittal and transaxial SPECT images. Planar bone scans also should be obtained. Positive bone scan findings usually need to be correlated with X-ray studies.

■ High resolution collimation improves the anatomical detail of both planar and SPECT bone scans. For high resolution pediatric bone scanning, a pinhole rather than a straight bore collimator may provide optimal anatomical detail.

**Figure 2.14**

Normal right **(a)** and left **(b)** lateral planar and transaxial SPECT **(c)** bone scans of the TMJ (straight arrows) in an asymptomatic adult. When interpreting SPECT images of the TMJ, the intensity of tracer uptake at the site is compared with the adjacent calvarium. Incidentally noted on the transaxial SPECT image is increased activity in the alveolar ridge of the maxilla due to recent dental extractions (curved arrow); an abnormal TMJ will often equal or exceed this degree of abnormal tracer uptake.

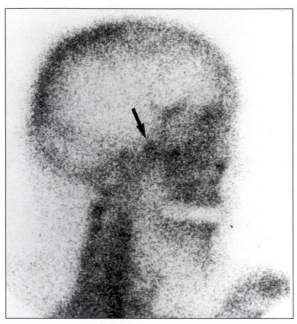

a

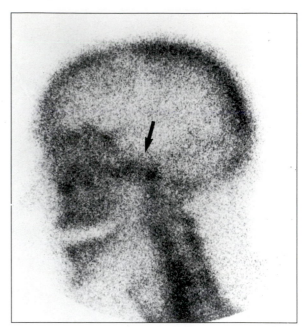

b

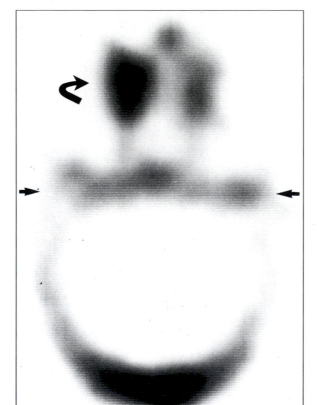

c

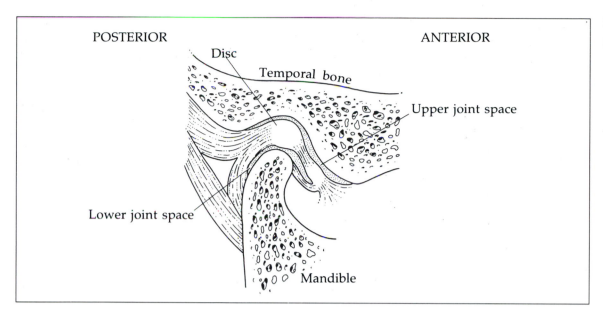

**Figure 2.15**
Sagittal view of the TMJ.

# ■ Teaching points

■

By eliminating activity surrounding the tomographic plane of interest, SPECT improves image contrast and provides additional useful anatomical information.

■

A normal SPECT bone scan should ideally show perfect left-to-right symmetry of all skeletal structures. In clinical practice this rarely happens. When positioning a patient for a SPECT study, even a slight degree of rotation or tilt results in SPECT images with left-to-right asymmetries. Practitioners must learn to distinguish skeletal pathology from these common errors in patient positioning. This often requires careful study of all three orthogonal (coronal, sagittal and transaxial) sets of SPECT images.

# Variants

## Skull sutures

**Figure 2.16 (a–c)**

Three examples of tracer uptake in skull sutures. It is common to see a focal area of increased tracer uptake which corresponds to the pterion, the site of confluence of the frontal, parietal, temporal and sphenoid bones. However, tracer uptake may be seen extending along individual sutures.

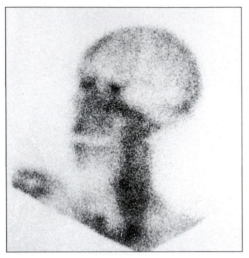

a

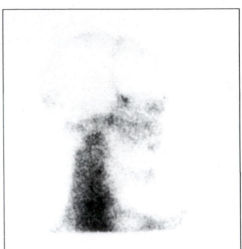

b

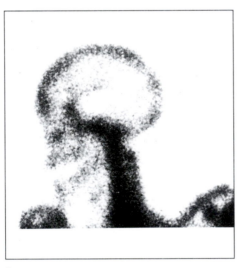

c

# Hyperostosis frontalis

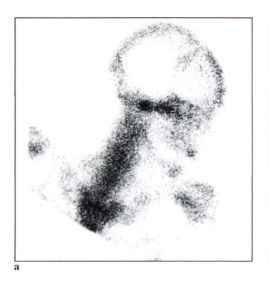

a

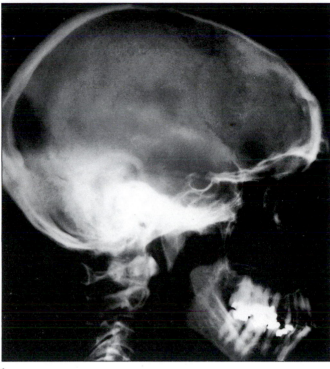

b

**Figure 2.17**

In elderly subjects, increased tracer uptake may be seen in the frontal region of the skull **(a)**, and these appearances are typical of hyperostosis frontalis. If clinically relevant, the diagnosis will be confirmed on a skull X-ray **(b)**.

# Occipital protuberance

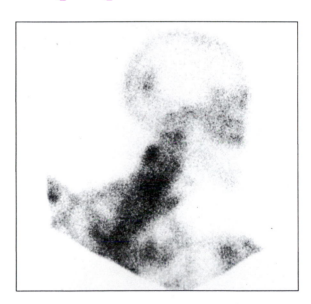

**Figure 2.18**

The skull is slightly rotated and a focal area of increased uptake is seen in the occipital region. This is a normal variant and corresponds to tracer uptake at the site of the occipital protuberance. Of course, coexistent pathology at this site cannot be absolutely excluded and, if clinically relevant, an X-ray may be required for further evaluation. Note that in this case there is a focus of increased uptake in the mid-cervical spine. This is a common finding and is most often due to degenerative change.

# Thyroid cartilage

**Figure 2.19**

An example of diphosphonate uptake in the thyroid cartilage. The uptake is thought to be due to microcalcification in the cartilage, and this finding is of no clinical relevance.

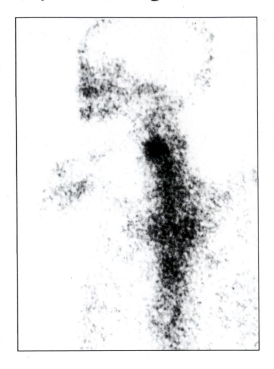

# Costochondral calcification

**Figure 2.20**

Tracer uptake is seen in the region of the costal cartilages. This is an extreme example, but may be seen in elderly subjects and is thought to be due to calcification of the cartilages.

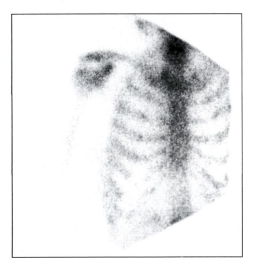

# Vascular calcification

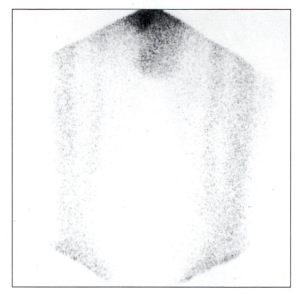

a

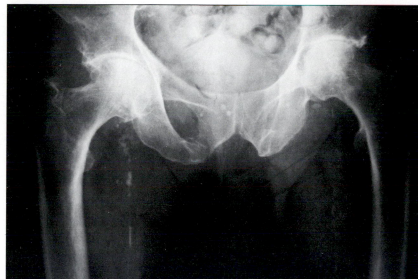

b

**Figure 2.21**

**(a)** Bone scan view of femora; **(b)** X-ray. Vascular calcification is apparent on the X-ray and there is corresponding uptake of tracer on the scan image.

# Tracer uptake at angle of Louis

**Figure 2.22**

There is a focal area of increased tracer uptake in the upper third of the sternum, between the manubrium and the body of the sternum. This is a common normal variant.

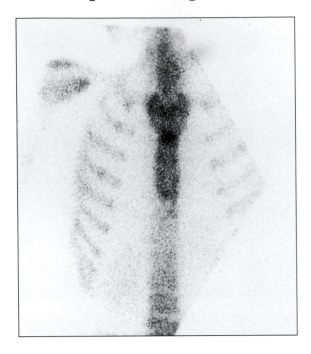

# Sternoclavicular uptake

**Figure 2.23**

Degenerative disease involving sternoclavicular joints. Focally increased tracer uptake is seen in the region of both sternoclavicular joints due to degenerative disease. While more pronounced than usual, this pattern of uptake is often seen and is of no clinical significance.

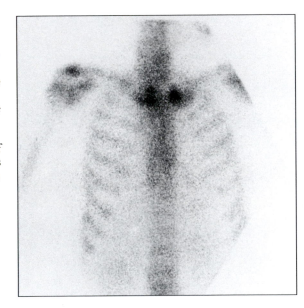

## Shine-through

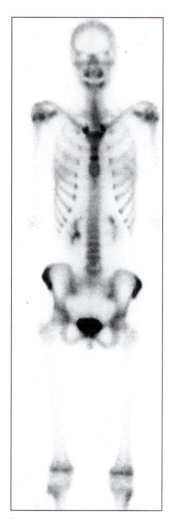
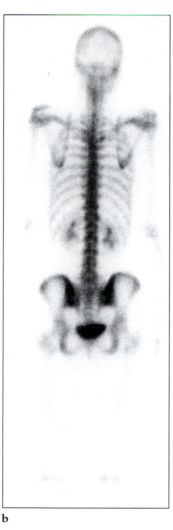

a          b

**Figure 2.24**

Normal **(a)** anterior and **(b)** posterior bone scans of a 16-year-old woman. On the anterior view prominent but normal tracer uptake is seen at the articulations of the clavicles with the manubrium and across the mid-sternum. On the posterior view, in which the patient is slightly rotated to the right, an apparent lesion is seen which represents 'shine-through' from the anterior end of the right clavicle.

## ■ Teaching point

■
When unable to distinguish 'shine-through' from a true rib lesion on a straight posterior view bone scan, obtain a posterior oblique view. A true lesion will remain in the same anatomical position within the rib while 'shine-through' will either change in position or disappear.

# Stippled ribs

**Figure 2.25**

Posterior view of the thoracic spine. Prominent activity is seen in the posterior aspect of multiple ribs. This appearance of so-called 'stippled ribs' is a normal variant, thought to be due to increased tracer uptake at sites of muscle insertion.

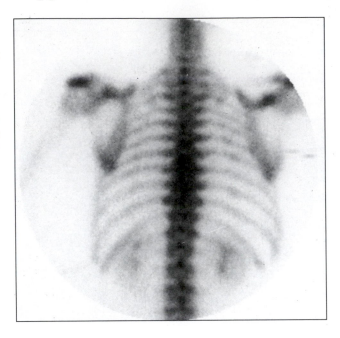

# 'Hot' patella sign

**Figure 2.26**

There is increased tracer uptake throughout both patellae, the so-called hot patella sign. For asymptomatic patients this finding should be considered a normal variant.

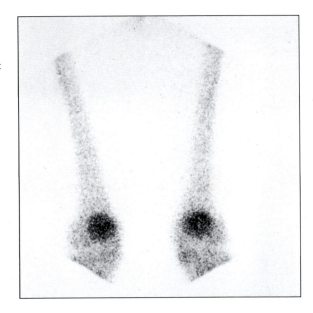

# Deltoid sign

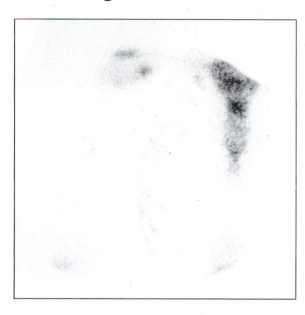

**Figure 2.27**

A focal area of increased tracer uptake is seen at the upper third of the right humerus. This corresponds to the deltoid tuberosity and the site of insertion of the deltoid muscle. It should be considered a normal variant; however, when it is pronounced, the physician should be alert to the possibility of coexistent disease, particularly if the patient is known to have a primary malignancy.

# Breast uptake

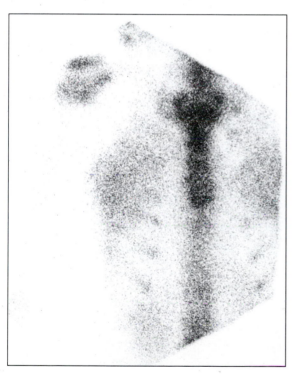

**Figure 2.28**

Bone scan view of the anterior chest of a 36-year-old woman. There is tracer uptake in both breasts; there was no explanation for this. The patient was not lactating, was not on medication and the breasts were normal to palpation.

# Spina bifida

**Figure 2.29**

Bone scan views: **(a)** posterior lumbar spine and **(b)** anterior pelvis; **(c)** X–ray of lower lumbar spine/pelvis. There is a small photon–deficient area associated with the L5/S1 region which, on the X–ray, is attributable to the incomplete partial fusion of the spinous processes.

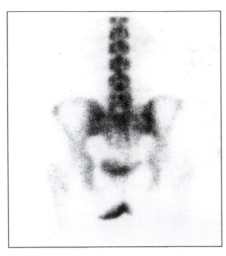

a

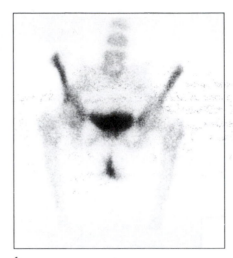

b

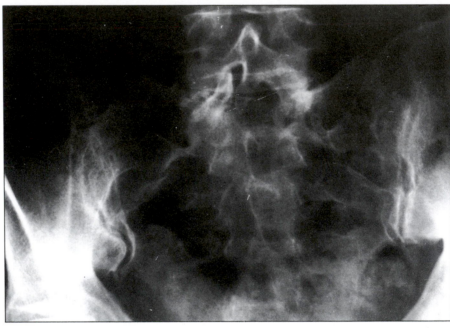

c

# Large lumbar transverse processes

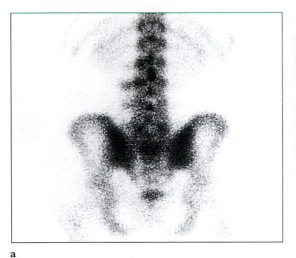

a

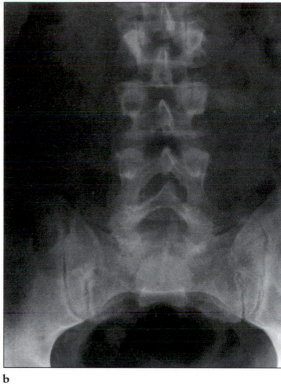

b

**Figure 2.30**

(a) Bone scan view, posterior lumbar spine; (b) X-ray. There is increased tracer uptake associated with the left transverse processes of L3 and L4, in keeping with the developmental abnormality noted on X-ray.

# Sacralization of 5th lumbar vertebra

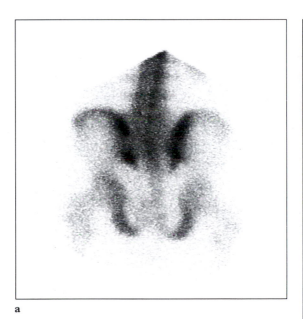

a

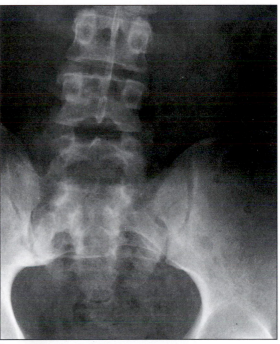

b

**Figure 2.31**

The posterior view bone scan of the pelvis and lower lumbar spine (a) shows striking asymmetry between the two sacroiliac joints, with less marked difference in tracer uptake over the two sides of the 5th lumbar vertebra. The X-ray (b) demonstrates a normal variant adequate to account for the asymmetries on the bone scan. There is so-called 'sacralization' of a large left-sided transverse process of L5, with associated bony changes in the sacrum.

# Dental disease

**Figure 2.32**

A focus of increased tracer uptake is seen at the angle of the left mandible. Focal abnormalities in the mandible and maxilla are common and most often reflect dental disease. In this case, the patient had an apical abscess. If clinically relevant, however, an X-ray may be required for further evaluation because, although it is an extremely rare occurrence, patients can present with a solitary metastasis at this site (see page 106).

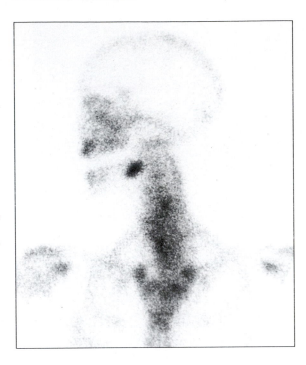

# Pelvic kidney

**Figure 2.33**

Bone scan views: **(a)** posterior lumbar spine and **(b)** anterior pelvis. On the posterior view, the right kidney is not visualized and increased tracer uptake is seen in the region of the right sacroiliac joint. The anterior view, however, clarifies these findings, and there is a right-sided pelvic kidney which is contributing to the 'shine-through' seen on the posterior view. In this case there is also increased tracer uptake in the left hip, which is due to degenerative disease.

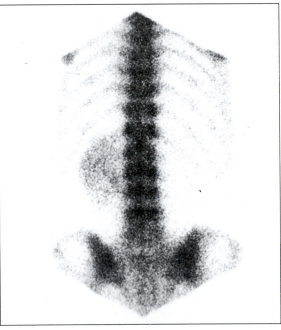

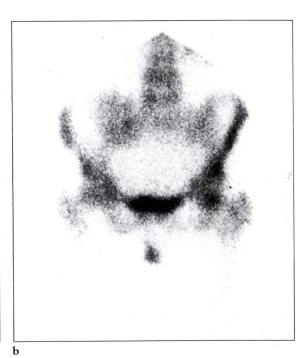

a

b

# Artefacts and pitfalls

## Urine contamination

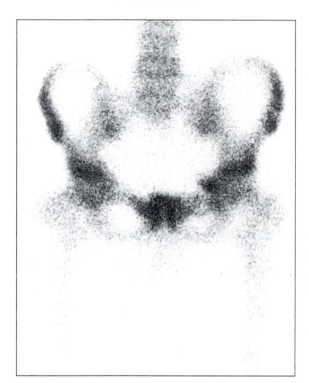

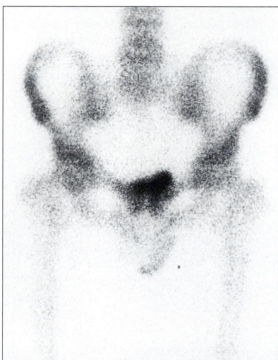

a

b

**Figure 2.34**
Bone scan views of anterior pelvis. A focal area of increased tracer uptake is seen medial to the left acetabulum **(a)**. This does not appear to be in bone and is caused by urine contamination. The repeat study **(b)** was normal.

## Uptake in central venous line

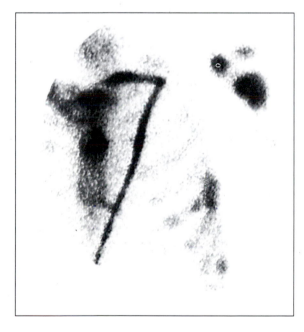

**Figure 2.35**
$^{99m}$Tc-MDP injection via a Hickman catheter in a patient with metastatic breast carcinoma. Intense activity is seen adhering to the catheter. This intense activity persisted after flushing the catheter with a saline bolus.

---

## ■ Teaching point

---

■
$^{99m}$Tc-MDP and many other commonly used radiopharmaceuticals will adhere to plastic catheters.

---

# Activity at site of injection

**Figure 2.36**

A right-sided injection has been tissued. Note that an axillary lymph node is visualized on that side (arrow). There is no clinical significance associated with this finding.

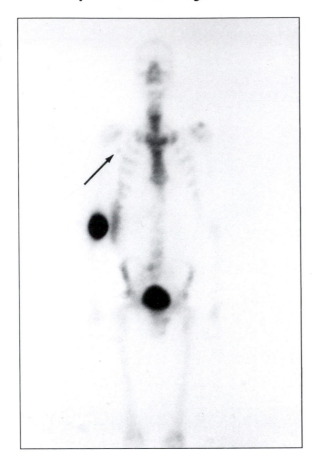

# Previous radionuclide administration

**Figure 2.37**

On the bone scan image there is massive increased tracer accumulation in the neck. This was due to a therapeutic dose of $^{131}I$, which the patient had received 2 weeks earlier for toxic multinodular goitre. The 364 keV photon from $^{131}I$ will penetrate the septa of a low energy collimator causing distortion of the image. In this case a medium energy collimator was used to obtain the image.

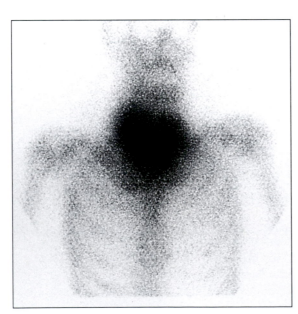

# Free pertechnetate

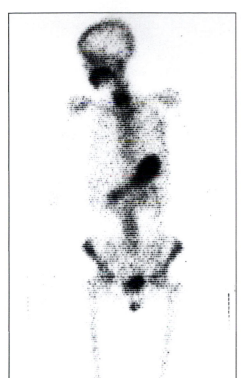

**Figure 2.38**

Tracer uptake is seen in the mouth, salivary glands, thyroid and stomach. These are the typical appearances found in the presence of free pertechnetate.

# The importance of correct contrast

**Figure 2.39**

Two case where the focal nature of a lesion was not apparent from analogue images. **(a, c)** Analogue. **(b, d)** Digital. In both cases, at higher contrast, generally increased tracer uptake is visualized at the site of abnormality. However, at lower contrast, the discrete nature of the lesions is apparent.

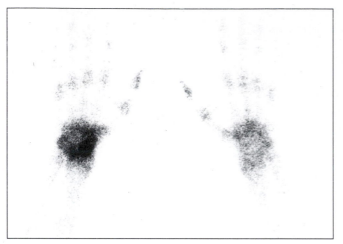

a

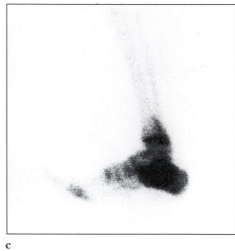

c

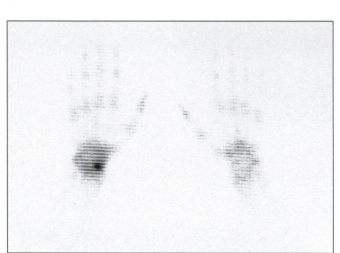

b

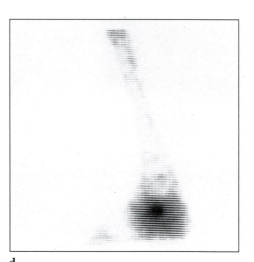

d

---

# ■ Teaching point

---

■

If digital images are obtained, then the data can be reviewed and the contrast altered if necessary. With analogue images, the correct contrast has to be obtained at the outset, and if the quality of images is inadequate then the study has to be repeated.

# Artefacts

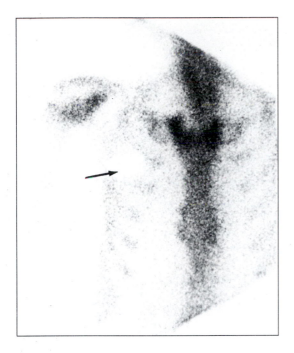

**Figure 2.40**

Artefact (arrow) caused
by a pacemaker.

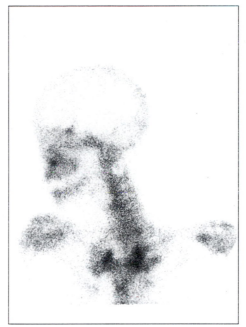

**Figure 2.41**

Artefact caused by
earrings.

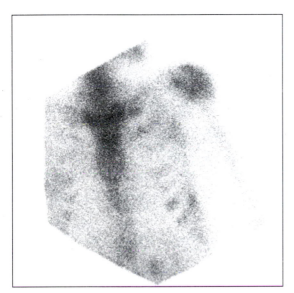

a

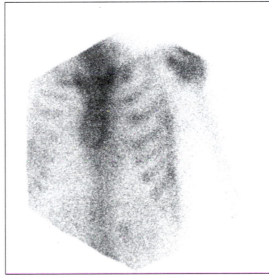

b

**Figure 2.42**

Artefact caused by a breast
prosthesis. Note that there
is a relatively photon-
deficient area overlying
the left anterior chest **(a)**
due to the breast
prosthesis. The repeat
image with the breast
prosthesis removed **(b)** is
normal.

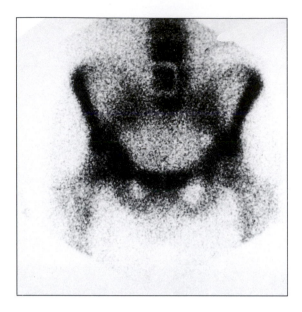

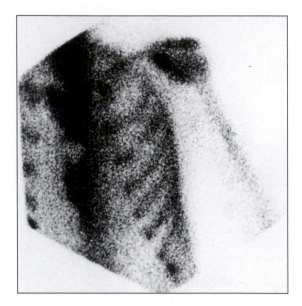

**Figure 2.43**

Artefact caused by a belt buckle.

**Figure 2.44**

Artefact caused by a medallion.

**Figure 2.45**

Barium in the rectum. Bone scan views: **(a)** posterior pelvis, and **(b)** lateral pelvis. There is a photon-deficient area posterior to the bladder, corresponding to the rectum. This patient had a barium meal examination 1 week previously, which was the cause of the photon-deficient area.

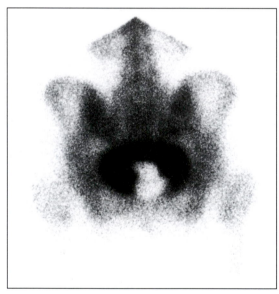

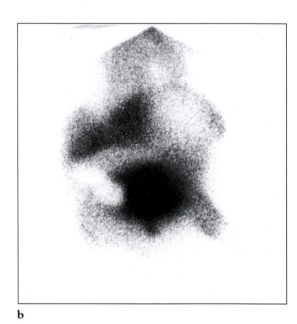

a

b

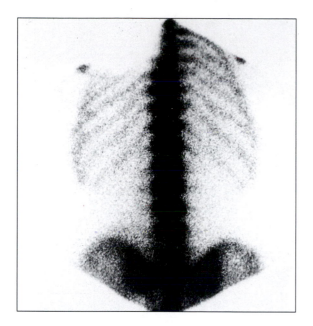

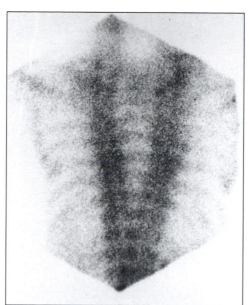

**Figure 2.46**

There is a photon-deficient lesion in the upper right of the image, due to a photomultiplier tube defect.

**Figure 2.47**

Motion artefact.

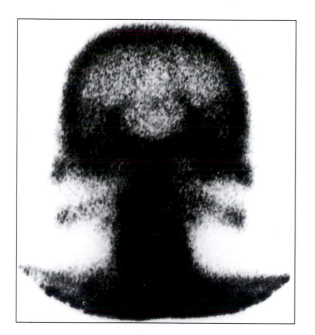

**Figure 2.48**

Superimposition of right and left lateral views of skull.

# SPECT artefacts and pitfalls

**Figure 2.49**

Normal coronal SPECT bone scan **(a)** in a young adult volunteer with slight left-to-right asymmetries caused by scoliosis, which are most marked in the SIJ region. The presence of scoliosis often makes SPECT studies of the spine difficult to interpret. The planar bone scan **(b)** shows the scoliotic curve to better advantage.

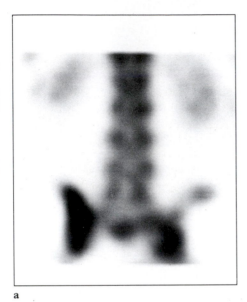
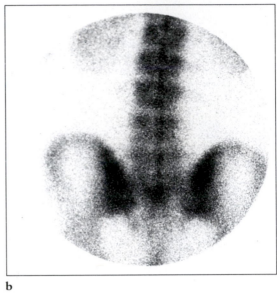

a                                                                b

**Figure 2.50**

A low count SPECT was acquired at 2 seconds per projection rather than the normal 20 seconds per projection. Note the 'grainy' appearance due to inadequate counting statistics.

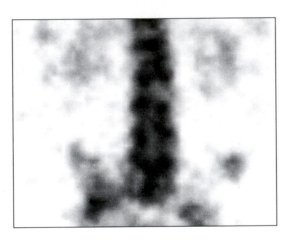

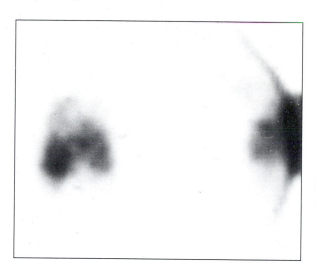

**Figure 2.51**

SPECT data was intentionally acquired with the left knee partially outside the field of view when the camera was in front and behind the volunteer. The resulting transaxial SPECT bone scan shows the typical 'in and out of field of view' artefact; this is a type of incomplete angular sampling artefact.

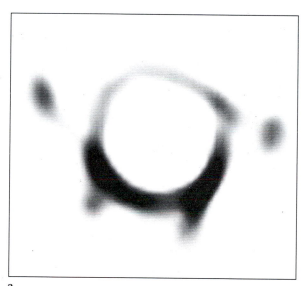

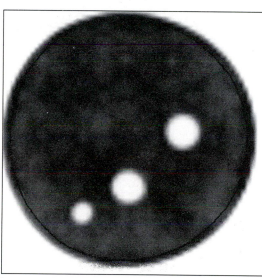

**Figure 2.52**

The 'hot' ring artefact on a transaxial bone SPECT image **(a)** may be produced when there are 'cold' spots on the uniformity flood. In clinical practice such artefacts are rarely encountered on SPECT bone scans. This artefact was produced by placing three lead circles on an otherwise uniform $^{57}$Co sheet source and then acquiring an 'incorrect' uniformity correction flood **(b)**.

a                                    b

**Figure 2.53**

A transaxial SPECT image of the pelvis obtained as a patient's bladder filled rapidly during the time of SPECT data acquisition. Broad rays project beyond the bladder and obscure bony pelvic structures. The increase in bladder counts between the beginning and the end of gamma camera rotation creates this artefact. Either bladder catheterization or imaging at 6 rather than 2–3 hours following injection can eliminate this artefact. The bladder-filling artefact is a type of incomplete angular sampling artefact.

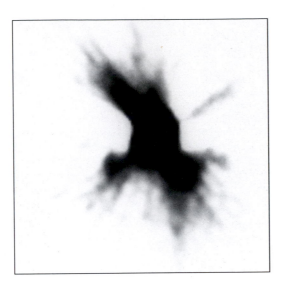

# Metastases

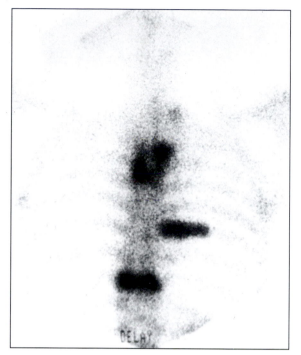

a

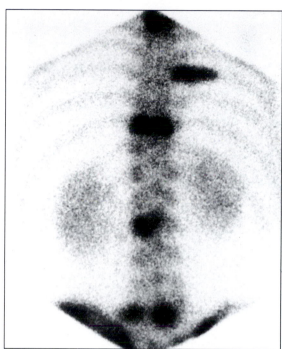

b

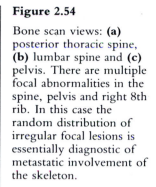

**Figure 2.54**

Bone scan views: **(a)** posterior thoracic spine, **(b)** lumbar spine and **(c)** pelvis. There are multiple focal abnormalities in the spine, pelvis and right 8th rib. In this case the random distribution of irregular focal lesions is essentially diagnostic of metastatic involvement of the skeleton.

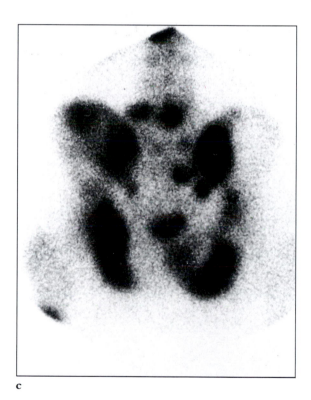

c

**Figure 2.55 (a–g)**

Carcinoma of the breast, with more extensive involvement of the skeleton. Virtually every bone appears abnormal and, in additon to focal lesions, there is marked irregularity of tracer uptake in the ribs; such appearances should always alert the physician to the possibility of metastatic involvement. Note that the appearance of the humeral and femoral heads is grossly abnormal, which usually reflects extensive marrow disease.

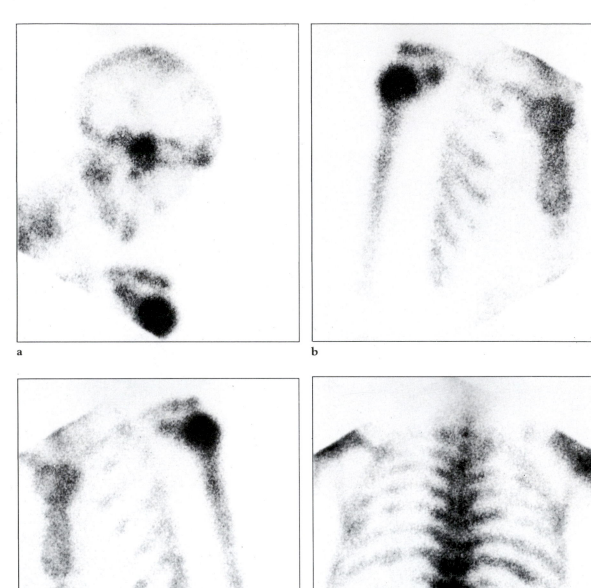

a

b

c

d

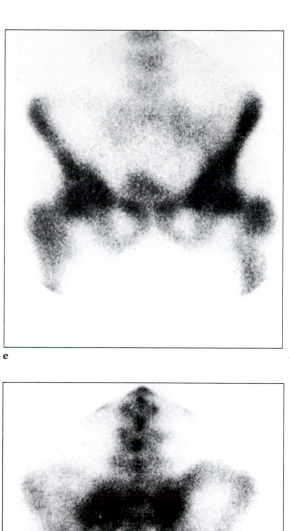

e

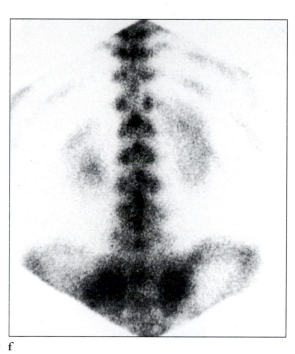

f

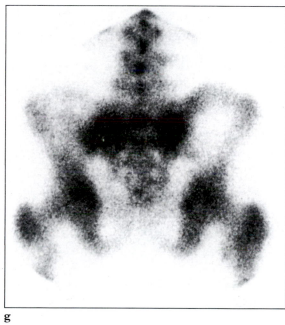

g

# 'Superscan' of malignancy

A 'superscan' may be defined as a bone scan where there is increased and relatively uniform tracer uptake throughout the skeleton, with high contrast between bone and soft tissues. Renal images will either be faintly visualized or not seen, because of increased contrast between bone and kidneys. In addition, high uptake of tracer by the skeleton leaves less available for excretion via the urinary tract.

**Figure 2.56**

The 'superscan' of malignancy **(a–g)**. There is such extensive involvement of the skeleton by tumour that individual lesions have coalesced. In such cases patchy uptake of tracer is usually seen, particularly in the ribs, with occasional more focal lesions. Note that the kidneys are not visualized. If any doubt exists as to whether the bone scan is normal or abnormal, a single X-ray of the pelvis **(h)** will clarify the issue. Sclerotic metastases are seen throughout all bones.

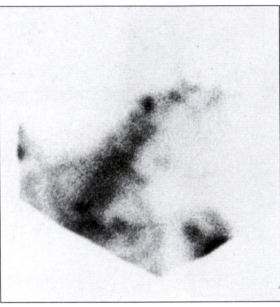

a

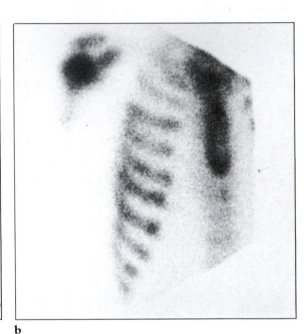

b

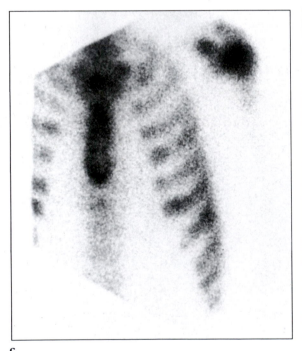

c

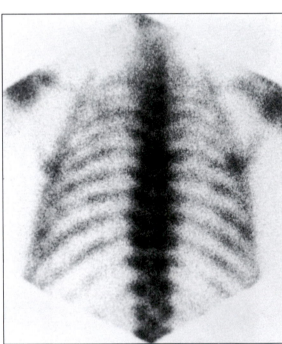

d

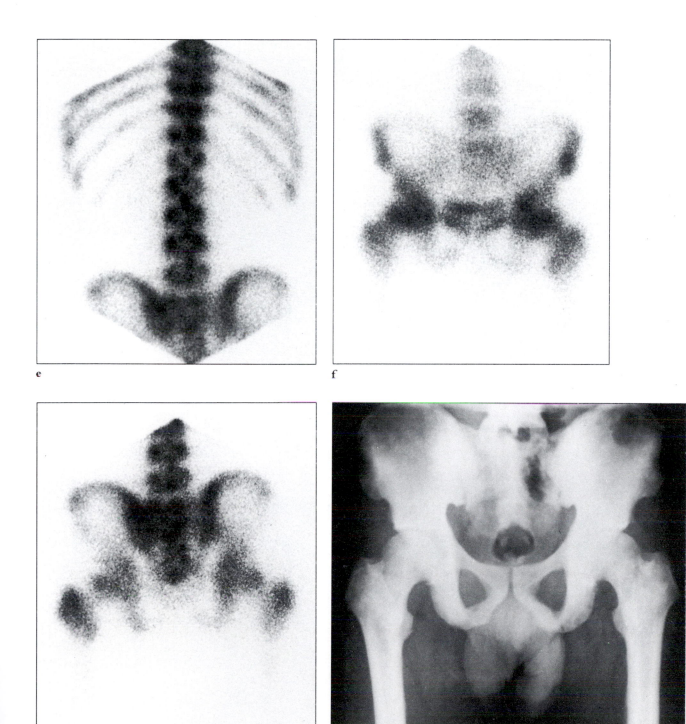

e

f

g

h

### Table 2.1 The 'superscan'

| Causes | Helpful features |
| --- | --- |
| Malignancy | Irregularity of tracer uptake |
| | Focal lesions |
| | Often skull and long bones poorly visualized |
| Hyperparathyroidism | Metabolic features |
| | Hypercalcaemia |
| Osteomalacia | Metabolic features |
| | Pseudofractures |
| Delayed imaging in normal subject | Usually requires more than 6 hour delay |

**Figure 2.57**

A further example of the 'superscan' of malignancy where scan appearances are much more difficult to evaluate. Bone scan views: **(a)** anterior and **(b)** posterior. There is high uptake of tracer throughout the axial skeleton, with the kidneys only faintly visualized, but there is also increased tracer uptake in the skull and long bones – features shared with metabolic bone disease. However, there is also more focally increased tracer uptake in the left shoulder, and uptake in the region of the left anterior superior iliac spine is slightly irregular.

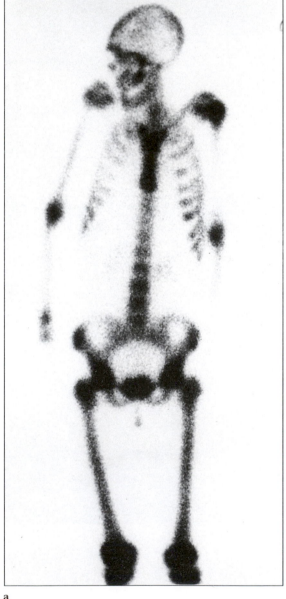

a

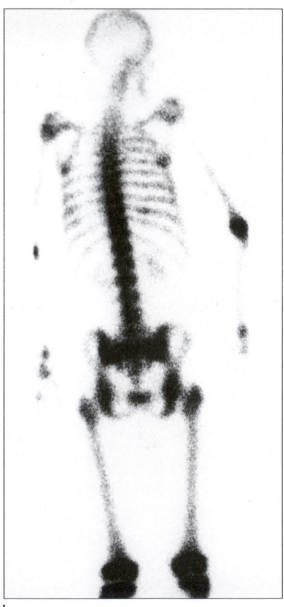

b

# Hypertrophic pulmonary osteoarthropathy

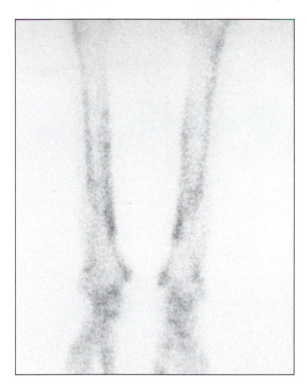

**Figure 2.58**
Bone scan view of tibiae, showing increased tracer uptake, particularly associated with the cortical margins. The scan findings are typical of hypertrophic pulmonary osteoarthropathy in association with carcinoma of the lungs. This is a good example of the so-called tramline or parallel stripe sign.

# Marrow hyperplasia

**Figure 2.59**

A 23-year-old woman with sickle cell disease. Bone scan views: **(a)** anterior chest, **(b)** anterior pelvis and **(c)** lower limbs. There is symmetrically increased tracer uptake at the ends of the long bones. The scan findings are typical of hyperactive marrow.

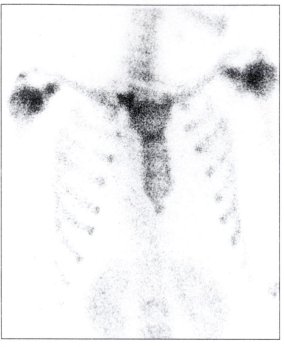

a

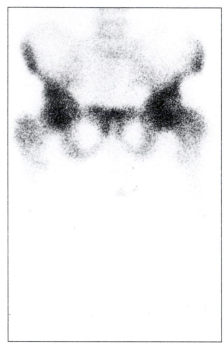

b

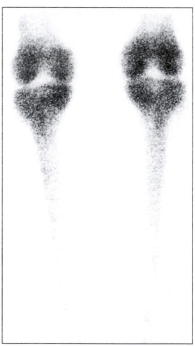

c

# Trauma

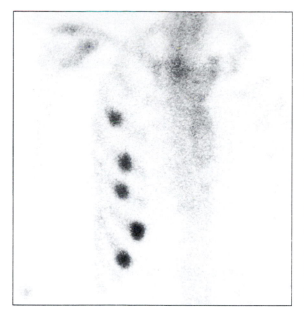

a

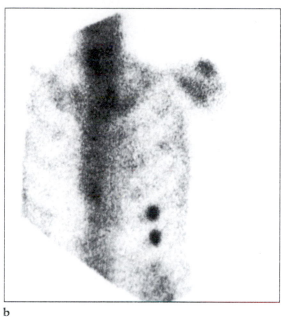

b

**Figure 2.60 (a, b)**

Two cases with focal abnormalities present in the ribs anteriorly. The linear pattern is typical of rib fractures one above another in adjacent ribs. This linear pattern of lesions in short segments of rib is not seen with malignancy (compare with Figure 2.61).

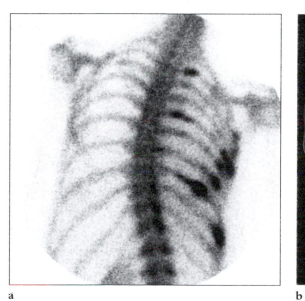

a

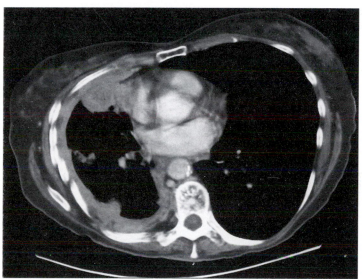

b

**Figure 2.61**

A 54-year-old man with pleural mesothelioma and chest wall invasion. The bone scan image **(a)** shows multiple lesions in the ribs, many of which are in a linear pattern. However, most of the lesions show extension along the rib. In particular, many of the lesions seen on the posterior view bone scan involve longer segments of rib than typically occurs with simple fractures. The CT scan **(b)** in this patient previously thought to have benign pleural thickening, shows evidence of chest wall invasion. Subsequent chest-wall biopsy provided the histologic diagnosis.

# ■ Teaching points

■

A linear pattern of 'clustered' focal rib lesions 2 cm or less in length are characteristic of fractures, while lesions involving longer segments of rib are suspicious for malignancy.

■

Fractures often occur in characteristic patterns that can be recognized on bone scan.

1 *Rib fractures* usually involve short focal lesions in multiple adjacent ribs.

2 *Pelvic fractures* usually involve at least two sites of the bony pelvic ring. For example, sacroiliac joint diastasis often occurs in association with fractures of the superior and inferior pubic rami (see Figures 5.31 and 6.34).

3 *Fractures of osteoporotic vertebra* usually appear as bands of increased uptake extending horizontally across the vertebral bodies. Adjacent vertebral body end plates may be involved (see Figures 2.66–2.68).

4 *Mid-foot fracture dislocations* frequently involve the tarsometatarsal joints (see Figures 5.33 and 5.34).

# Arthritis

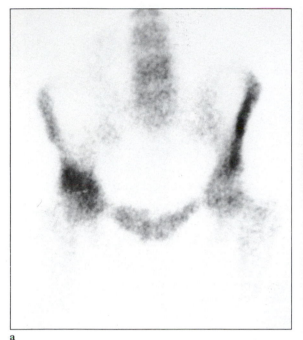

a

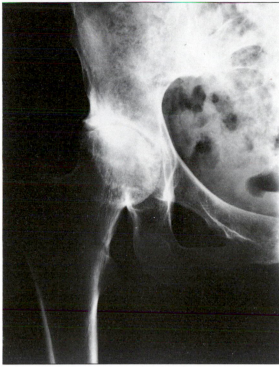

b

**Figure 2.62**

A bone scan view of the anterior pelvis **(a)** shows increased tracer uptake in the region of the right hip. Such a finding in isolation is most often due to arthritis, which is confirmed in this case on the X-ray **(b)**.

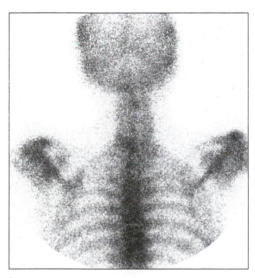

a

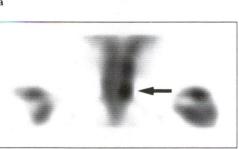

b

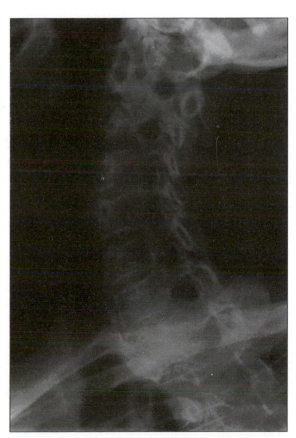

c

**Figure 2.63**

A focal area of increased tracer uptake is seen to the left of the mid-line in the lower cervical spine on a posterior view planar bone scan **(a)**. The finding is more convincingly demonstrated and better localized on a coronal SPECT bone scan image **(b)** (arrow). The X-ray **(c)** confirms osteoarthritis at the left-sided C6–C7 Luschka joint.

**Figure 2.64**

In this case there is a focal area of increased tracer uptake in the left 1st carpometacarpal joint **(a)**. The scan findings are typical of osteoarthritis at that site, and this is confirmed on the X-ray **(b)**.

a

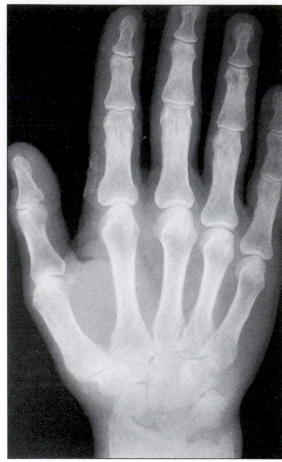

b

# Metabolic bone disease

■ **Metabolic features present on bone scan:**

1 High tracer uptake in axial skeleton
2 High tracer uptake in long bones
3 High tracer uptake in periarticular areas
4 Faint or absent kidney images
5 Prominent calvaria and mandible
6 'Beading' of the costochondral junctions
7 'Tie' sternum

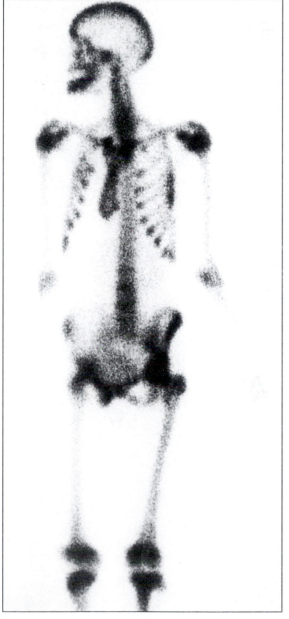

a

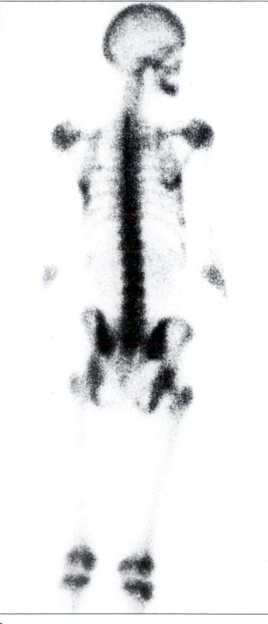

b

**Figure 2.65**

A 21-year-old woman with anorexia nervosa and osteomalacia. Bone scan views: **(a)** anterior and **(b)** posterior. There is a strikingly increased tracer uptake present throughout the skeleton, with high contrast between bone and soft tissue. The renal images are not visualized. Note, in addition, the high uptake of tracer in the calvaria and mandible in keeping with hyperparathyroidism. 'Beading' of the costochondral junctions and a 'tie' sternum are also present. All of these features are characteristic of metabolic bone disease. The high uptake of tracer at the ends of the long bones is somewhat unusual and may represent epiphyseal uptake, reflecting delayed maturation of the skeleton.

# Vertebral collapse

**Figure 2.66**

Posterior bone scan view of the lumbar spine and pelvis of a 77-year-old woman with severe osteoporosis and vertebral collapse. There are two linear areas of increased tracer uptake involving L2 and L3. The appearances are typical of vertebral collapse.

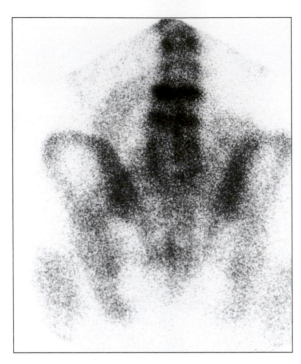

**Figure 2.67**

Posterior bone scan view of the lumbar spine. There is an intense linear area of increased tracer uptake in L1, due to benign vertebral collapse.

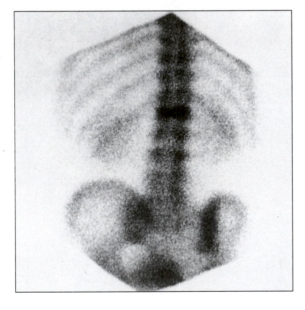

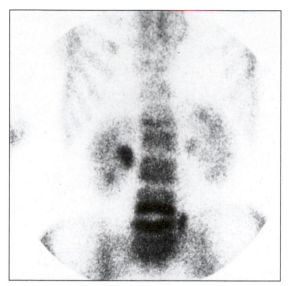

a

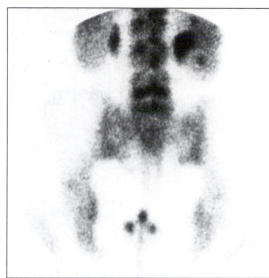

b

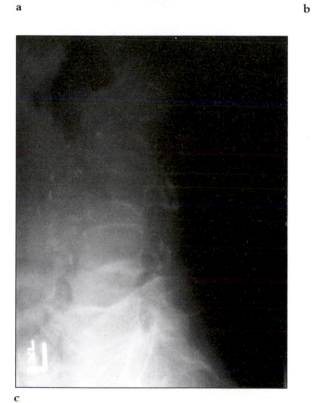

c

**Figure 2.68**

Acute L4–L5 vertebral body endplate fractures in an osteoporotic 72-year-old woman. Anterior (a) and posterior (b) view bone scans show prominent tracer uptake, which is best explained by recent fractures. Axial loading of the lumbar spine probably caused herniation of the nucleus pulposus through these adjacent vertebral body end plates. The X-ray (c) shows advanced osteoporosis and multiple lumbar vertebral body fractures. The older vertebral fractures show little or no increased tracer uptake.

## Discitis

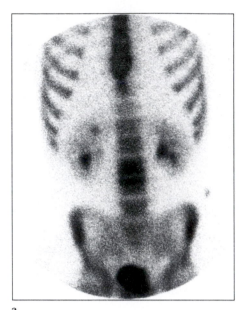

a

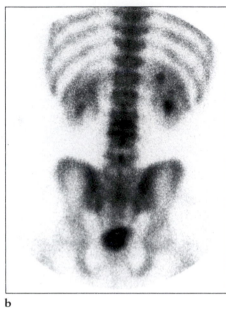

b

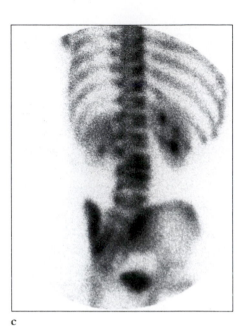

c

**Figure 2.69**

Aspergillus discitis in a 32-year-old male iv drug abuser. There is intense increased tracer uptake at the vertebral body end plates adjacent to the L2–L3 intervertebral disc space on the anterior **(a)**, posterior **(b)** and RPO **(c)** planar bone scan images. Less pronounced increased tracer uptake is seen deep within the L2 and L3 vertebral bodies. Coronal plane SPECT bone scan images **(d)** localize the process to the vertebral bodies but fail to resolve the intervertebral disc space. While unlikely in this age group, a similar scan appearance could be produced by herniation of the nucleus pulposus into adjacent vertebral body end plates.

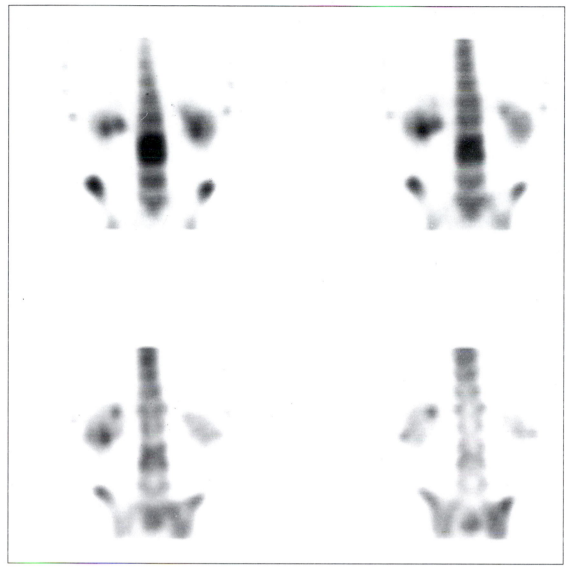

d

## ■ Teaching point

■
The 'typical' appearance of vertebral body endplate fractures may be mimicked by discitis. Radiographic correlation or even aspiration biopsy may be necessary.

# Paget's disease

**Figure 2.70**

Intense uptake of tracer is seen throughout the body of L3, which appears 'expanded'. Note that the transverse processes are clearly visualized. The scan findings **(a)** are typical of Paget's disease. There is also increased tracer uptake in the sacrum, presumably also reflecting pagetic involvement. The X–ray **(b)** confirms Paget's disease involving L3, but appearances in the sacrum were thought to be normal.

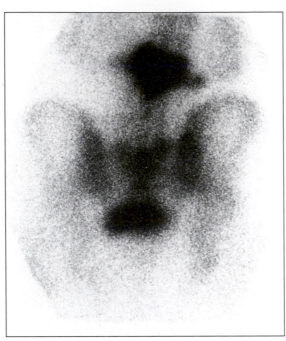

a

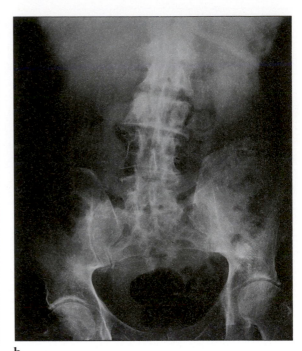

b

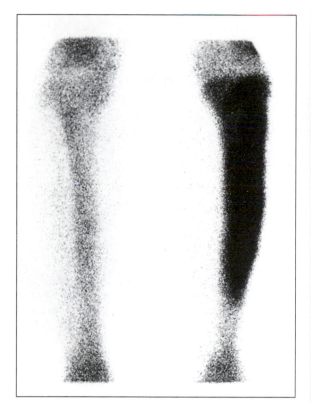

a

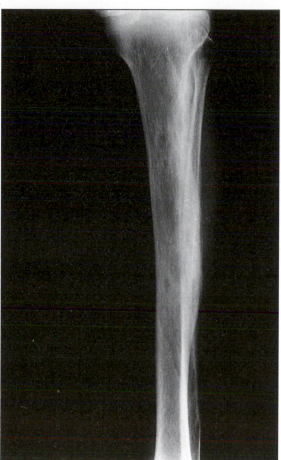

b

**Figure 2.71**
A further example of Paget's disease. There is strikingly increased tracer uptake involving most of the left tibia. The scan appearances **(a)** are typical of Paget's disease, which is confirmed on the X–ray **(b)**.

## ■ Teaching point

■ Paget's disease of the tibia or other long bones is characterized by extension from the diaphysis all the way to the end of the bone.

# Clinical indication for bone scanning: investigation of bone pain

3

The bone scan is widely used in clinical practice and is the most commonly requested investigation in any nuclear medicine department because of its sensitivity for lesion detection. The indications for a bone scan are continually being extended, but fall into three main categories:

- Investigation of bone pain (Chapter 3)
- Investigation of malignancy (Chapter 4)
- Investigation of benign bone disease (Chapter 5)

Clinical indications for bone scanning in patients with unexplained skeletal pain include the following:

- Metastasis
- Benign bone tumour
- Trauma and sports injuries
- Avascular necrosis and bone infarction
- Infection
- Osteomalacia
- Paget's disease
- Incidental findings

# Metastasis

**Figure 3.1**

A 76-year-old woman who complained of back pain. The bone scan shows increased tracer uptake in L1 (arrow), which is more pronounced on the left lateral border. There is no other skeletal abnormality present. An X-ray of the lumbar spine showed minor degenerative changes only. Biopsy of L1 was carried out, and tumour was identified. This patient did not have a known primary malignancy. In this case, there is a single focal abnormality present, and a metastasis cannot be diagnosed on the basis of the scan alone.

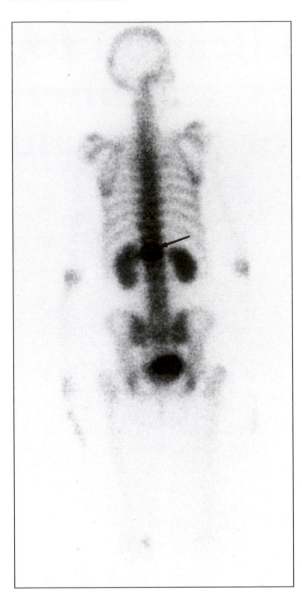

# Benign bone tumour

## Osteoid osteoma

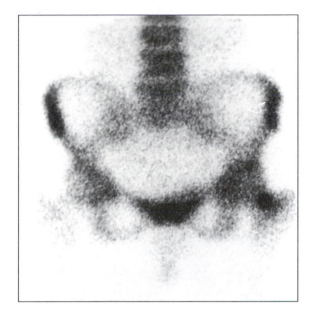

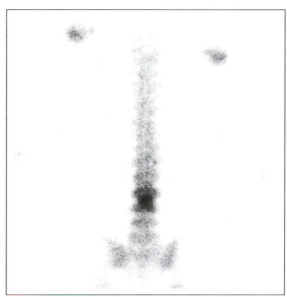

**Figure 3.2**

A 14-year-old boy who complained of pain in the left hip. The bone scan view of the anterior pelvis shows a discrete focus of strikingly increased tracer uptake in the left femoral neck. The scan appearances are strongly suggestive of osteoid osteoma: this was confirmed at surgery. The X-rays were normal.

**Figure 3.3**

A 6-year-old boy who complained of back pain. X-rays identified a lesion at L2, the nature of which was uncertain. The bone scan shows an intense discrete focus of increased tracer uptake at that site, an appearance which is strongly suggestive of osteoid osteoma. This was confirmed at surgery.

# Trauma and sports injuries

**Figure 3.4**

A 66-year-old woman who complained of pain in her anterior chest, caused by a fall while getting out of the bath. The bone scan view of the anterior chest shows marked linearly increased tracer uptake in the mid-sternum with further focal abnormalities present in the right 3rd and 4th, and left 3rd ribs anteriorly, close to the costochondral junctions. The scan findings are typical of fracture at the above sites.

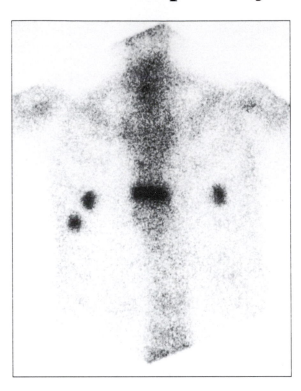

**Figure 3.5**

A 50-year-old man who had fallen on to his outstretched hand and was experiencing tenderness over the anatomical snuff-box area. Although a scaphoid fracture was clinically suspected, the X-ray **(a)** was thought to be normal. The bone scan **(b)** clearly shows a focal bone lesion, typical of a scaphoid fracture.

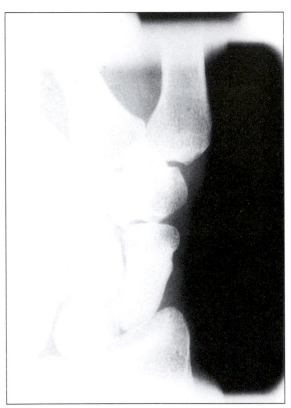

a

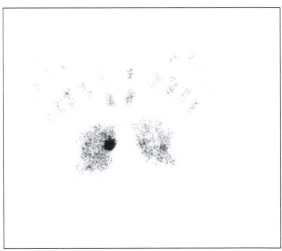

b

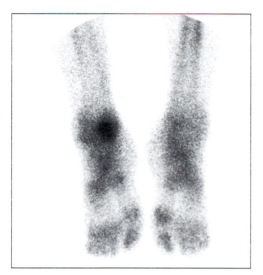

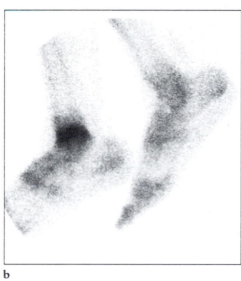

a

b

**Figure 3.6**

A 25-year-old man with persistent ankle pain following an inversion injury. Bone scan views of feet: **(a)** anterior and **(b)** lateral. Increased tracer uptake is seen over the medial aspect of the dome of the talus. The X-ray **(c)** shows a lucent lesion with a slightly sclerotic margin at this site, typical of a transchondral fracture. Osteochrondritis dissecans can have the same bone scan and X-ray findings.

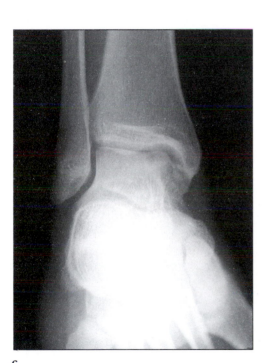

c

**Figure 3.7**

A case of osteochondritis dissecans. A 22-year-old man who complained of pain in his left ankle. Bone scan views of feet: **(a)** blood pool, **(b)** anterior and **(c)** lateral. Static images show a small intense focus of increased tracer uptake in the region of the medial aspect of the dome of the talus. This is vascular. The initial X-rays were normal. It was felt that the bone scan appearances were likely to be due to an osteoid osteoma, but at surgery a small defect in the posterior surface of the articular cartilage covering the talus was seen. The diagnosis was osteochondritis dissecans, related to a previous injury.

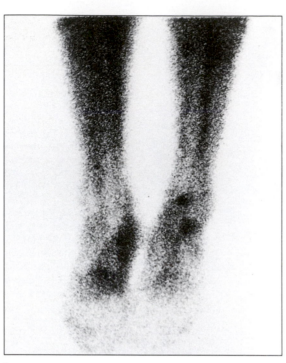

a

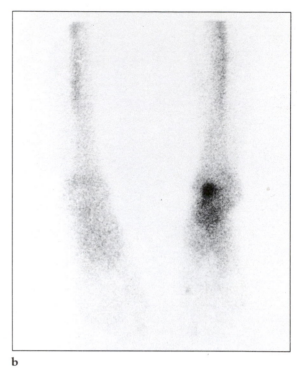

b

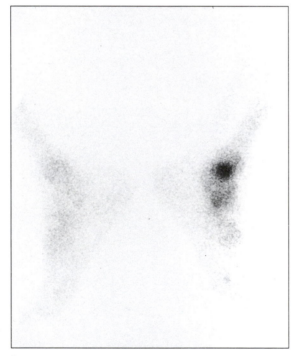

c

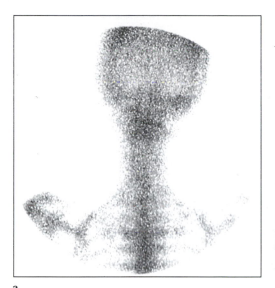

a

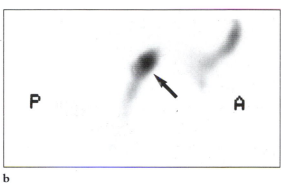

b

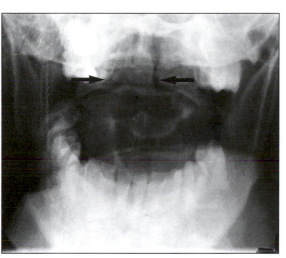

c

**Figure 3.8**

A 26-year-old woman with neck and back pain following an automobile accident. No convincing abnormality is seen on the posterior planar bone scan **(a)**. The mid-line sagittal SPECT image **(b)** shows increased activity in the upper cervical spine (arrow). The open-mouth X-ray **(c)** reveals a fracture of the odontoid process (arrows).

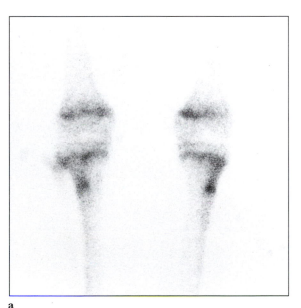

a

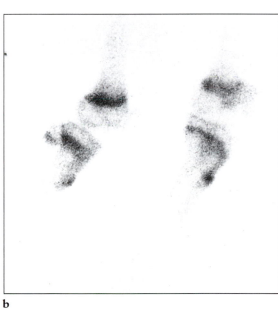

b

**Figure 3.9**

An 18-year-old man who complained of pain in his knees. Bone scan views of knees: **(a)** anterior and **(b)** lateral. There are symmetrical focal lesions just below, and lateral to, the tibial tuberosities. The scan findings are likely to represent small stress lesions, which are metabolically active and relate to the site of muscle insertion. The area of abnormality on the scan corresponded with the site of the patient's symptoms.

**Figure 3.10**

A 17-year-old ballet
dancer who complained of
pain in her lower left leg.
Bone scan views of lower
limbs: **(a)** blood pool, **(b)**
delayed anterior image
and **(c)** delayed lateral
image. There is a focus of
intensely increased tracer
uptake present at the
lower end of the left
fibula. This is vascular.
Although the initial X-
rays were normal, this
area corresponded to a
stress fracture seen on
subsequent X-rays.

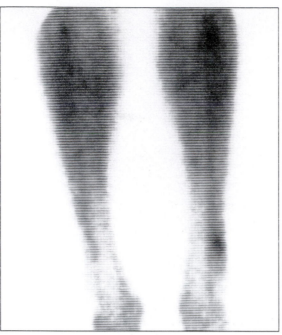

a

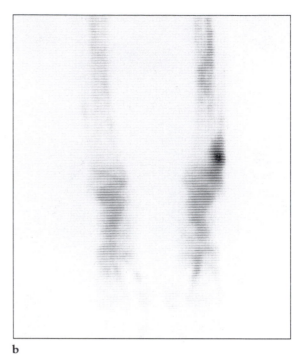

b

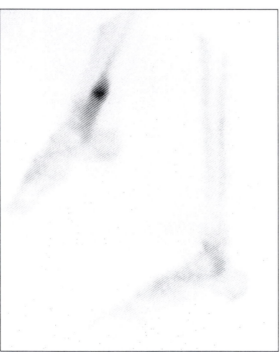

c

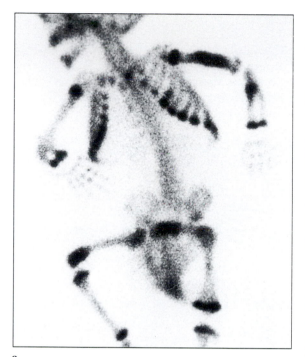

a

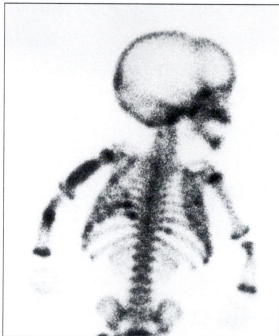

b

**Figure 3.11**

A 9-month-old male infant with bony tenderness. Bone scan views of skeleton: **(a)** anterior, **(b)** and **(c)** posterior. Focal abnormalities are present in the right 11th and left 9th and 10th ribs posteriorly, left 5th rib anteriorly, left humerus, left radius, left mid–femur and right knee. Thus there are multiple lesions throughout the skeleton, and the scan appearances are strongly suggestive of non-accidental injury.

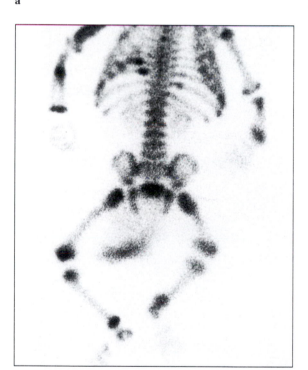

c

## ■ Teaching points

■

In non-accidental injury in infants, the bone scan may occasionally miss skull fractures, so a skull X-ray should be obtained routinely.

■

Sometimes, pinhole views of the epiphyses may be of value, as this is a common site of fracture; a lesion may not be apparent on the initial study.

# Reflex sympathetic dystrophy syndrome

The reflex sympathetic dystrophy syndrome is poorly understood, and is often forgotten in clinical practice. It is seen most commonly following trauma, and symptoms include pain and tenderness, swelling and dystrophic skin changes. Other terms applied to this syndrome include:

- Causalgia
- Acute atrophy of bone
- Sudeck's atrophy
- Post-traumatic osteoporosis
- Shoulder–hand syndrome

**Figure 3.12**

A 20-year-old man who continued to complain of pain in the right knee following an injury to that site. Bone scan views of knees: **(a)** dynamic, **(b)** blood pool and **(c)** anterior. The bone scan study shows diffusely increased tracer uptake associated with all three bones involving the knee joint. There is increased vascularity to the area. These findings are typical of reflex sympathetic dystrophy syndrome. Two arthroscopies were performed, which both gave negative results. The clinical diagnosis was one of reflex sympathetic dystrophy syndrome following trauma.

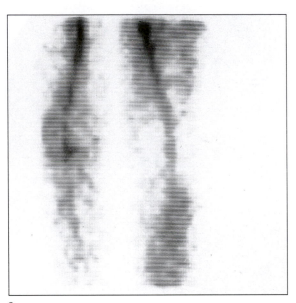

a

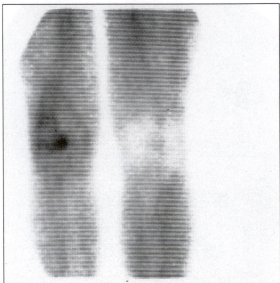

b

c

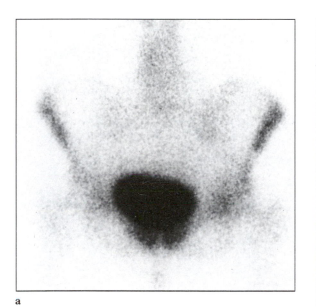

a

b

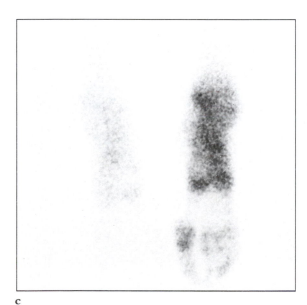

c

**Figure 3.13**

Bone scan views: **(a)** anterior pelvis, **(b)** femora and **(c)** feet. There is increased tracer uptake present in all the bones of the left leg, but it is most marked at the femoral neck, knee, ankle and forefoot. The scan findings are typical of reflex sympathetic dystrophy syndrome and are commonly seen in patients who have been immobilized, eg, following a stroke.

## ■ Teaching point

■

The reflex sympathetic dystrophy syndrome is easily recognized when it involves multiple joints of the hand or leg, all of which would be covered by a long glove or stocking.

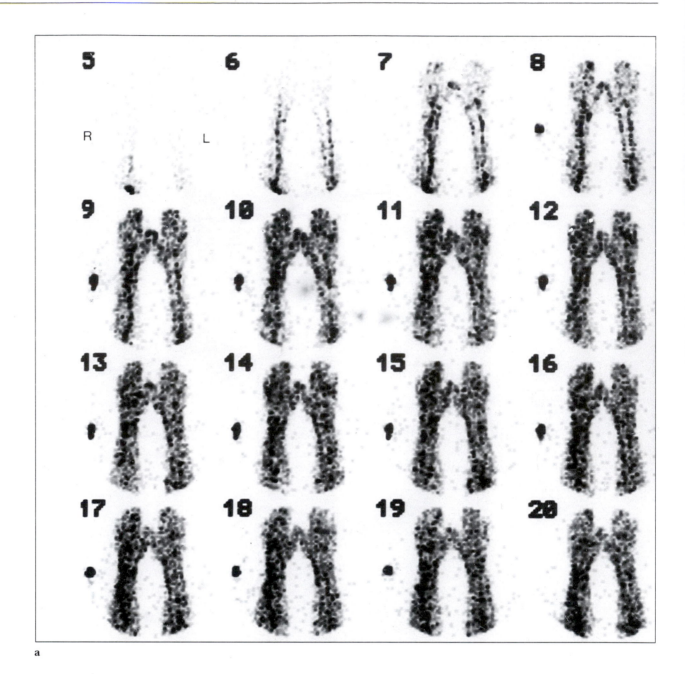

a

**Figure 3.14**

A 34-year-old woman with persistent left arm pain for 6 months following a fall. Bone scan views of forearms: **(a)** dynamic of hands and wrists, **(b)** hands and wrists, and **(c)** elbows. There is increased tracer uptake near the visualized joints of the left forearm. The diagnosis was that of reflex sympathetic dystrophy, and pain was relieved by stellate ganglion block. Note that typical scan findings are seen on the 3 hour delayed bone scan, but the dynamic study does not show increased vascularity in the left arm.

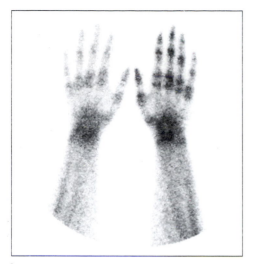

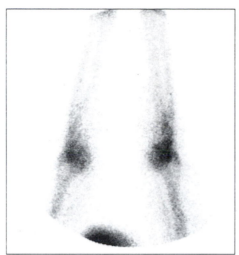

b                                        c

## ■ Teaching point

■
Although typically there is increased
vascularity, the reflex sympathetic
dystrophy syndrome may be present
even when dynamic and blood pool
scans are normal.

# Avascular necrosis and bone infarction

■ **Causes**

1 Trauma
2 Caisson disease
3 Sickle cell disease
4 Radiation
5 Vascular injury

6 Gaucher's disease
7 Steroid therapy
8 Idiopathic, eg, Legg–Perthes disease
9 Alcoholism
10 Pancreatitis

**Figure 3.15**

A case of avascular necrosis of the hips caused by steroid therapy. The bone scan shows increased tracer uptake in both hips, which is more pronounced on the left. This patient has a renal transplant, which is seen on the scan in the right iliac fossa.

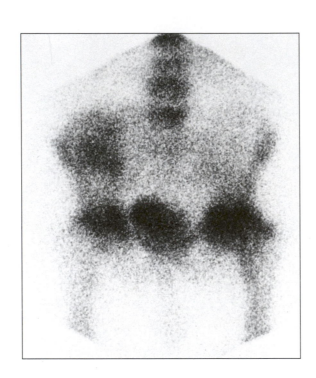

**Figure 3.16**

A 71-year-old woman with sickle cell disease who complained of pain in her left thigh. Bone scan views: **(a)** upper femora and **(b)** lower femora/upper tibiae. Several focal areas of increased tracer uptake are seen in the left upper and mid-femur. In addition, there is increased tracer uptake at the ends of the long bones. The scan appearances are those of multiple bone infarcts involving the left femur, together with marrow hyperplasia.

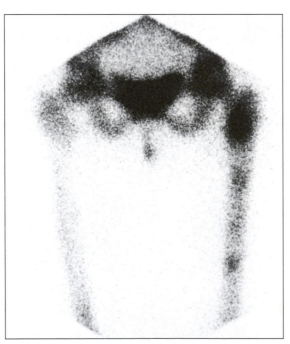

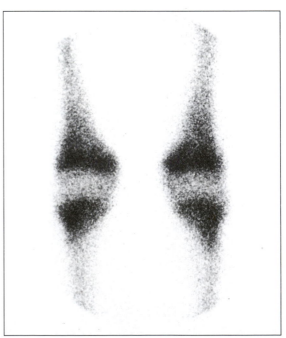

a

b

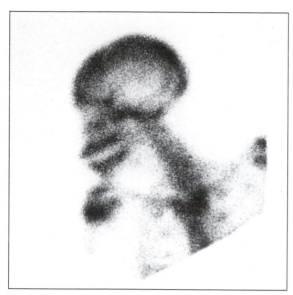

a

## Figure 3.17

A 30-year-old woman with sickle cell disease with bone and splenic infarcts. Bone scan views: **(a)** left lateral skull, **(b)** right anterior chest, **(c)** left anterior chest, **(d)** posterior thoracic spine, **(e)** posterior lumbar spine, **(f)** posterior pelvis, **(g)** anterior pelvis, **(h)** femora and **(i)** tibiae. X-rays: **(j)** pelvis and upper femora, and **(k)** femur. On bone scan views multiple focal abnormalities are present in the spine at T5 and T9, left 4th rib posteriorly, both femora and femoral heads, right upper tibia, both shoulders, right sternoclavicular joint and right 5th rib anteriorly. There is also tracer uptake diffusely throughout the spleen. There are extensive metabolically active lesions throughout the skeleton. This patient had severe sickle cell disease, and lesions represented bone infarcts **(j, k)**. Splenic uptake of tracer presumably reflects splenic infarction.

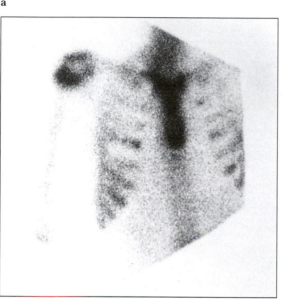

b

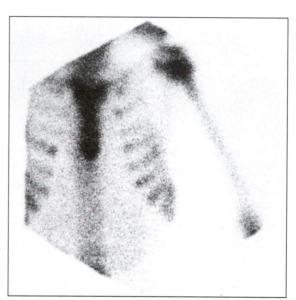

c

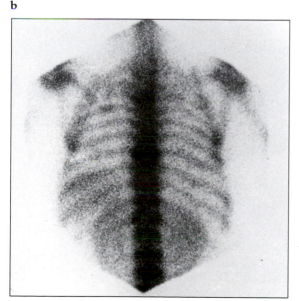

d

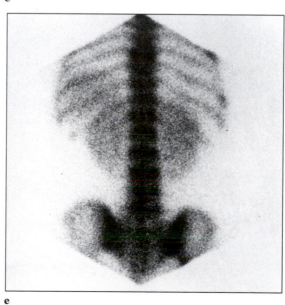

e

**Figure 3.17** *continued*

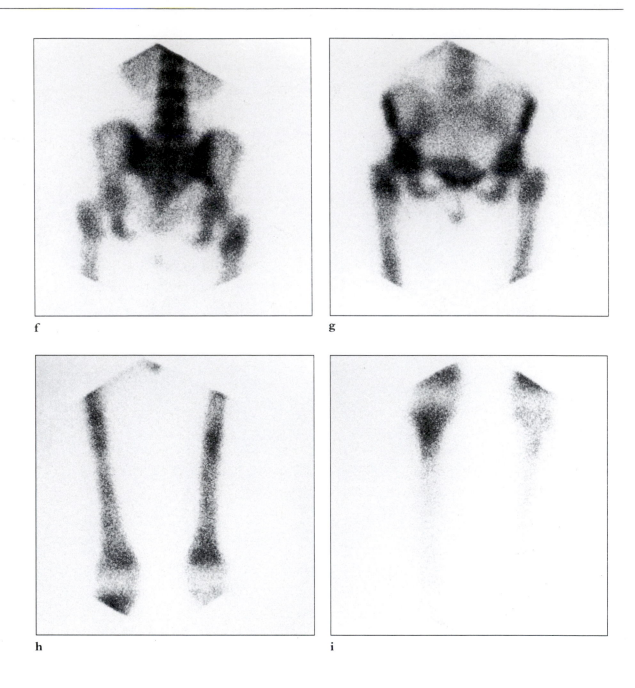

f

g

h

i

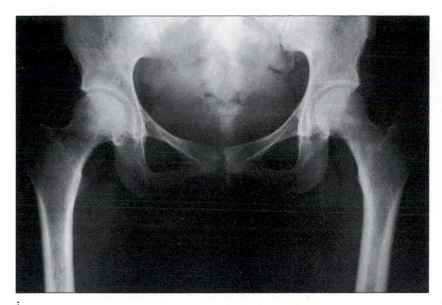

j

## ■ Teaching point

■
While avascular bone is represented by a photon–deficient area on a bone scan, in practice this may not be seen. A frequent finding is increased tracer uptake which reflects the healing response by surrounding bone.

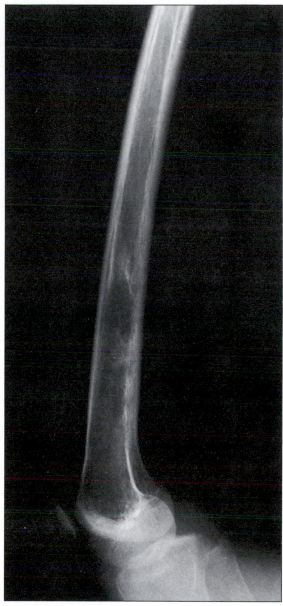

k

# Infection

**Figure 3.18**

An 18-year-old boy who presented with pain in the right tibia. Bone scan views of lower limbs: **(a)** dynamic, **(b)** blood pool, **(c)** anterior and **(d)** right lateral. There is a large vascular, metabolically active lesion present in the right upper tibia. At operation a Brodie's abscess (chronic, low-grade osteomyelitis) was found at that site.

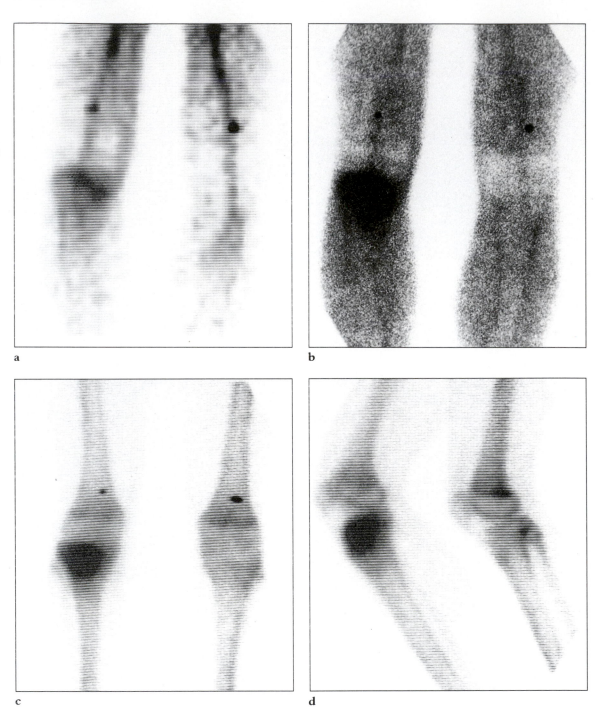

a

b

c

d

## ■ Teaching point

■

In the case shown in Figure 3.18, markers have been placed above the knees. These may help in the evaluation of a dynamic study, as it is frequently difficult to know if a vascular blush corresponds exactly to a metabolically active lesion.

# Osteomalacia

## ■ Causes

1 Poor exposure to ultraviolet light and low intake of dietary vitamin D
2 Vitamin D malabsorption, eg, coeliac disease
3 Abnormal vitamin D metabolism, eg, chronic renal failure
4 Peripheral resistance to vitamin D, eg, vitamin D-dependent rickets
5 Hypophosphataemia, eg, X-linked hypophosphataemic (or vitamin D-resistant) rickets
6 Hypophosphatasia
7 Inhibition of mineralization, eg, sodium fluoride

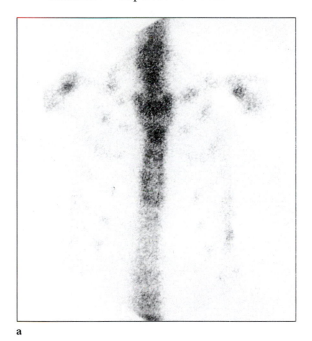

a

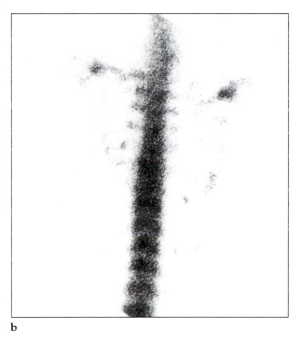

b

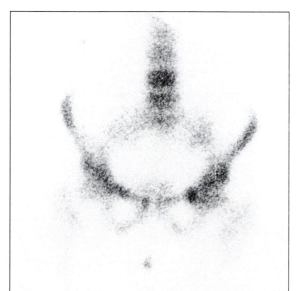

c

**Figure 3.19**

A 71-year-old woman who complained of generalized musculoskeletal pain. Bone scan views: **(a)** anterior chest, **(b)** posterior thoracic spine, and **(c)** anterior pelvis. The bone scan study shows generally good uptake of tracer throughout the skeleton, with high contrast between bone and soft tissue. There are multiple focal abnormalities in the ribs and left superior pubic ramus near to the acetabulum. This patient was shown to have osteomalacia with multiple pseudofractures.

## ■ Teaching point

■
The most common sites at which pseudofractures are seen on bone scan are:

| | |
|---|---|
| Ribs | 90% |
| Femur | 70% |
| Pelvis | 40% |
| Scapula | 20% |
| Forearm | 10% |
| Fibula | 10% |

# Paget's disease

**Figure 3.20**

A 61-year-old man who complained of low back pain. The bone scan shows strikingly increased tracer uptake throughout the whole of L5, and the bone appears expanded. No other abnormality was present throughout the skeleton. This patient had monostotic Paget's disease involving L5.

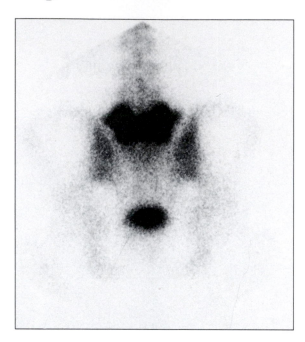

**Figure 3.21**

Incidence of Paget's disease on bone scans.

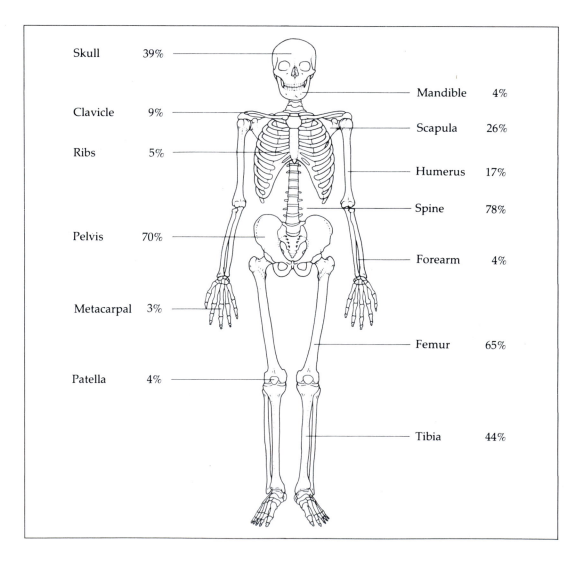

| Skull | 39% |
| Clavicle | 9% |
| Ribs | 5% |
| Pelvis | 70% |
| Metacarpal | 3% |
| Patella | 4% |

| Mandible | 4% |
| Scapula | 26% |
| Humerus | 17% |
| Spine | 78% |
| Forearm | 4% |
| Femur | 65% |
| Tibia | 44% |

# Incidental findings

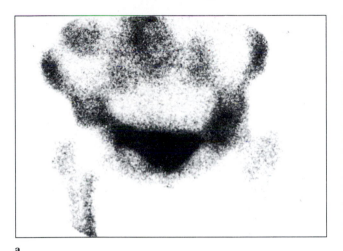

a

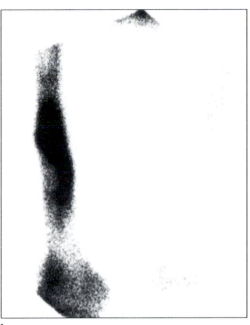

b

**Figure 3.22**

A 78-year-old woman who complained of pain in her right hip. Bone scan views: **(a)** anterior pelvis and **(b)** femora. She had had a total right hip replacement performed several years previously. The prosthesis is clearly identified on the bone scan, with no associated abnormality. However, there is strikingly increased tracer uptake in mid-shaft below the prosthesis, with the appearances suggestive of fracture. An X-ray confirmed spiral fracture at that site.

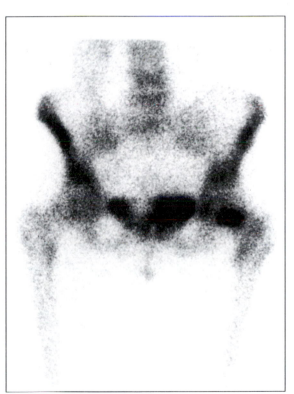

**Figure 3.23**

A 65-year-old woman who complained of pain in her left hip following a fall. The X-rays were normal, but the bone scan shows increased tracer uptake in the left femoral neck, with appearances suggestive of fracture. Subsequent X-rays confirmed an impacted fracture of the left femoral neck.

**Figure 3.24**

A 42-year-old woman who sustained trauma to her left forefoot. The X–rays were not thought to be typical of fracture and the possibility of primary bone tumour or infection was suggested. Bone scan views: **(a)** feet, **(b)** anterior thorax and **(c)** posterior lumbar spine. In addition to the abnormality in the left forefoot due to trauma, the scan appearances were thought to be strongly suggestive of metabolic bone disease. Although the patient felt well, with no other bone-related symptoms, biochemistry revealed chronic renal failure and significant renal osteodystrophy.

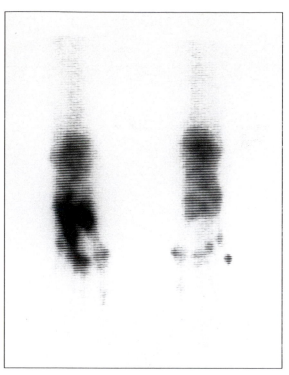

a

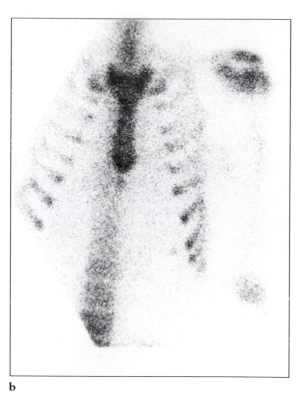

b

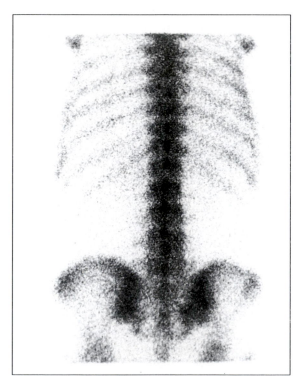

c

# Clinical indication for bone scanning: investigation of malignancy

- Initial staging
- Equivocal X-rays
- Assessment of the extent of disease
- Monitoring progress of disease and response to therapy
- Hypertrophic pulmonary osteoarthropathy
- Primary bone tumours

## Initial staging

The bone scan is important in the initial evaluation of patients with malignancy, as the knowledge that metastases are or are not present may alter subsequent management. The bone scan is extremely sensitive for lesion detection, and, in the case of carcinoma of the breast, when compared with routine radiography, has a lead time of up to 18 months (on average 4 months) for identification of metastases.

**Figure 4.1**

A 66-year-old man with carcinoma of the prostate. **(a)** Bone scan view of posterior pelvis; **(b)** X-ray of pelvis. On the bone scan there is markedly increased tracer uptake involving L5, with further focal abnormalities in the right ilium and right border of the sacrum. The scan appearances are those of metastatic disease, and this is confirmed on the X-ray.

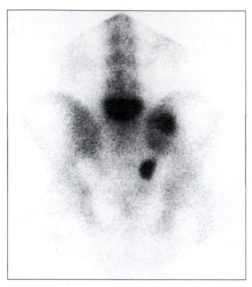

a

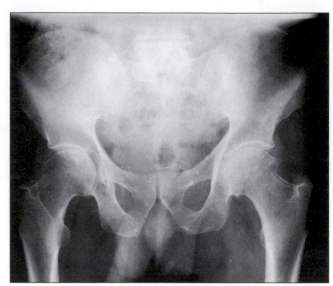

b

**Figure 4.2**

A further case of carcinoma of the prostate. Note that the bone scan appearances of the thoracic **(a)** and lumbar spine **(b)** are very abnormal, with multiple focal abnormalities throughout the skeleton. Renal images are not visualized. The scan appearances are approaching a 'superscan' of malignancy. However, in this case the X-rays were normal.

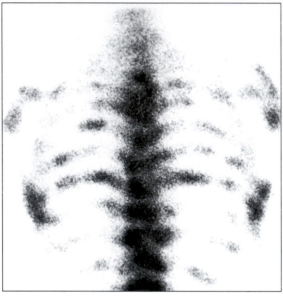

a

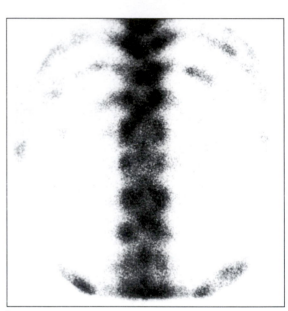

b

## Solitary metastasis in a rib

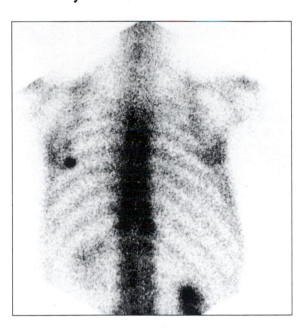

**Figure 4.3**

A patient with carcinoma of the breast who complained of pain in her back. The bone scan shows a focal area of increased tracer uptake in the right 7th rib posteriorly. No other abnormality is present. While a single, metabolically active lesion in a rib has only a 10 per cent probability of representing malignancy, in this case an X-ray of the area revealed a destructive lesion in the rib caused by a metastasis.

## Metastatic thyroid carcinoma

**Figure 4.4**

A 60-year-old woman who presented with left hip pain due to a metastasis from follicular carcinoma of the thyroid. Bone scan view: **(a)** posterior pelvis, **(b)** $^{131}$I view, posterior pelvis, **(c)** repeat bone scan view at time of $^{131}$I study; **(d)** X-ray of pelvis. The bone scan shows a focus of increased tracer uptake in the left iliac crest. There is probable abnormal tracer accumulation in the left sacroiliac joint extending into the sacrum. $^{131}$I scan shows avid tracer accumulation at the site of the iliac crest lesion but, in addition, there is tracer uptake at both sacroiliac joints, localization being confirmed by repeat bone scan at the time of the $^{131}$I study. The X-ray confirms the presence of metastatic disease.

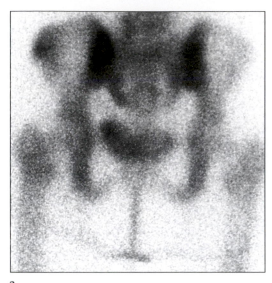

a

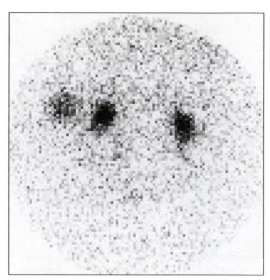

b

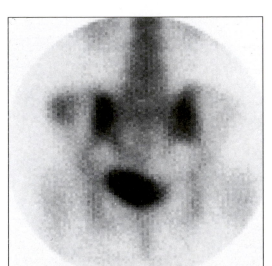

c

## ■ Teaching point

■

Abnormal $^{131}$I uptake in soft tissue or bone is highly specific for metastatic disease from well-differentiated thyroid carcinoma.

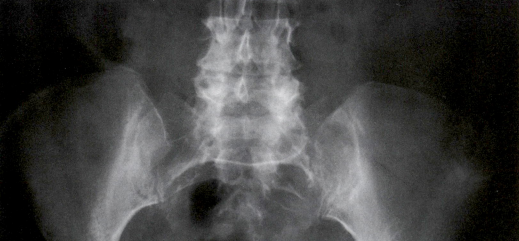

d

## Photopaenic lesion

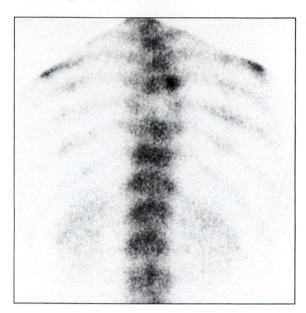

**Figure 4.5**

In this case of carcinoma of the lung, the bone scan shows a photon-deficient area at T9. In addition, there is a focal area of increased tracer uptake at the right border of T8 and there is generally patchy tracer uptake throughout the ribs. The scan appearances are those of metastatic disease.

## ■ Teaching point

■
While bone metastases usually produce increased tracer uptake, a small percentage of the skeletal metastases will produce photopaenic defects.

**Figure 4.6**

A 48-year-old man who complained of back and right leg pain. The posterior view bone scan of the pelvis **(a)** shows a curvilinear band of increased tracer uptake medially in the right ilium. Subsequent CT scan **(b)** identified metastatic lung carcinoma with extensive destruction of the right ilium. A magnified posterior view bone scan of the chest **(c)** shows another photopaenic metastasis, with increased activity limited to the bone at the margins of the tumour.

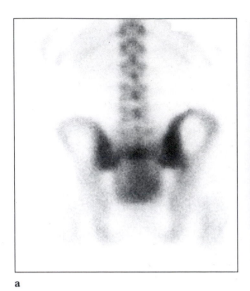

a

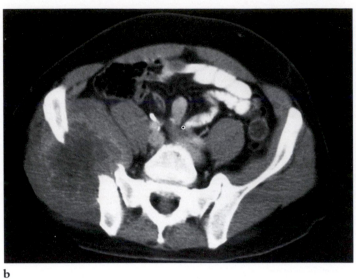

b

c

# ■ Teaching point

■
Although photopaenic lesions are relatively uncommon, it is important to identify them, as they usually indicate significant bony destruction. They may occasionally be seen in association with aggressive lytic disease, which does not induce an osteoblastic response.

## Recommended protocol for investigation of suspected skeletal metastases:

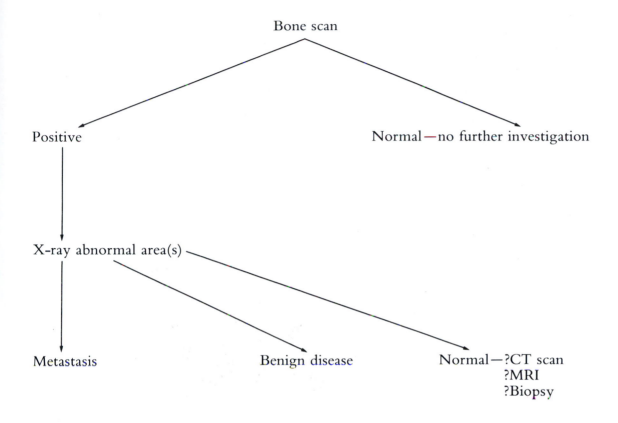

## Multiple myeloma

Multiple myeloma is the classic situation in which a false negative bone scan may be obtained. This occurs when the lesions are purely lytic, with no osteoblastic response. An example of this is shown in Figure 4.7, where the bone scan views appear essentially normal, but the X-rays show multiple lytic lesions throughout the skeleton. In practice, however, it is rare to see a completely normal bone scan in multiple myeloma when skeletal involvement is present.

**Figure 4.7 (a–k)**

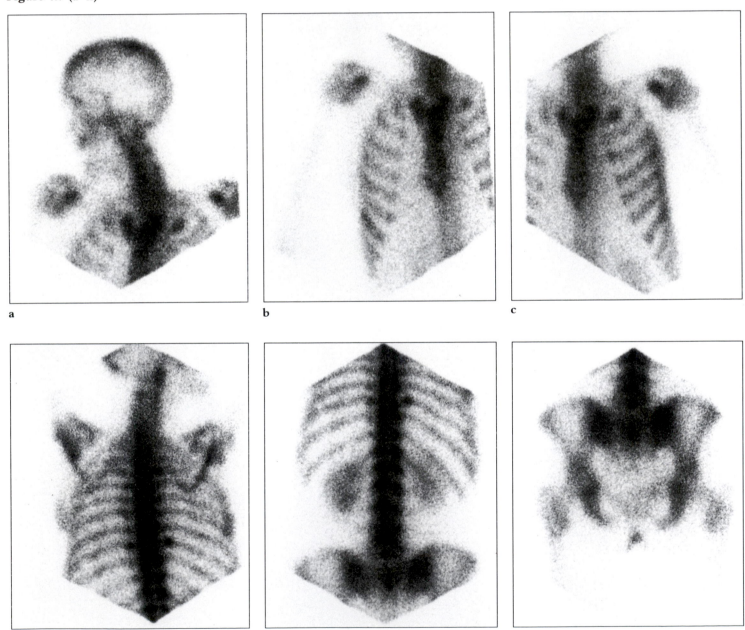

a

b

c

d

e

f

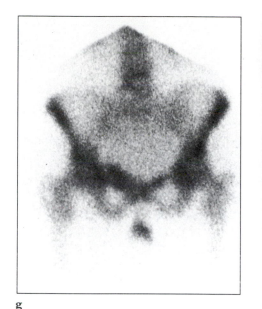

g

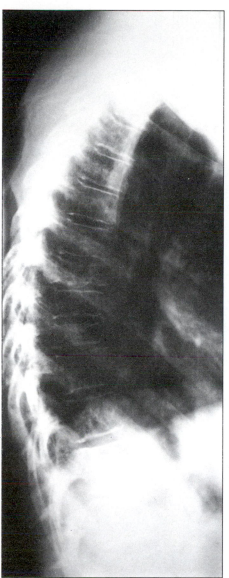

h

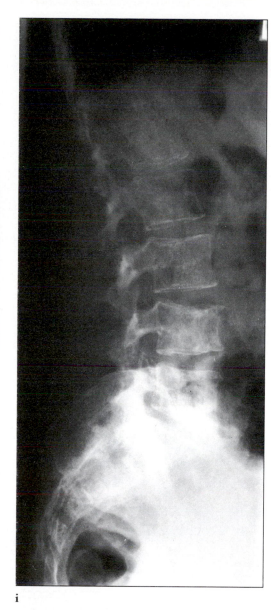

i

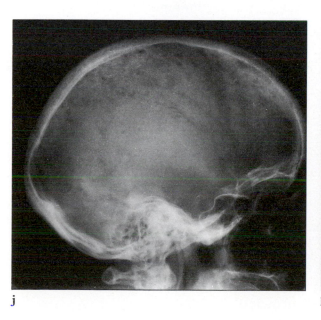

j

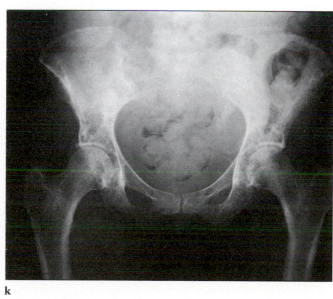

k

**Figure 4.8**

Two further cases of multiple myeloma.

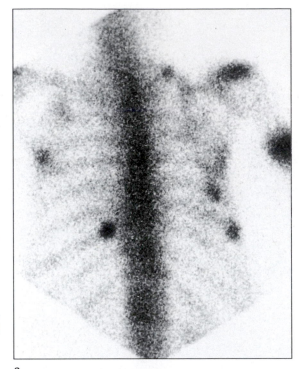

a

*Case 1:* **(a)** Several focal abnormalities are present throughout the ribs, with a large intense area of increased uptake in the mid-shaft of the right humerus. The scan findings represent bony involvement secondary to myeloma and pathological fracture of the right humerus.

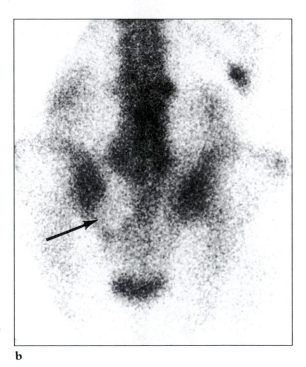

b

*Case 2:* **(b)** A large photon-deficient area is seen in the left border of the sacrum (arrow). In addition, focal areas of increased tracer uptake are present in the right 12th rib and L3.

## ■ Teaching point

■ While the bone scan may underestimate the extent of disease in multiple myeloma, it may, as in other situations, identify disease which is not apparent on X-rays. Radiography and bone scanning can be considered as complementary investigations when accurate documentation of all skeletal disease is required.

# Equivocal X-rays

## Solitary metastasis

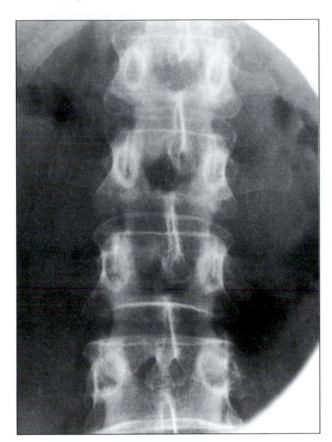

a

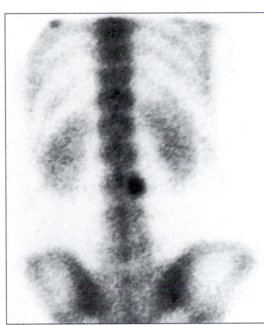

b

**Figure 4.9**

A patient with carcinoma of the breast who complained of severe low back pain. An X-ray **(a)** of the lumbar spine was normal. However, the bone scan **(b)** showed a discrete focal area of increased tracer uptake at the right border of L3. This was caused by a metastasis.

## Extensive metastases on scan with normal X-rays

**Figure 4.10**

A patient with carcinoma of the breast who had a bone scan for staging purposes. Multiple focal abnormalities representing metastases are seen throughout the skeleton (**a–c**). The radiographic skeletal survey (**d**) was normal at that time.

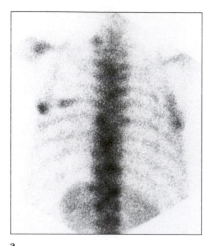

a

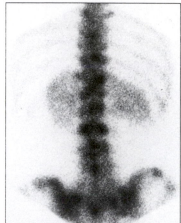

b

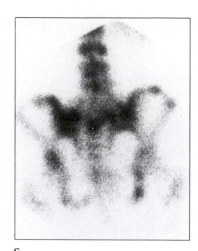

c

d

## ■ Teaching point

■
The bone scan may detect metastatic disease before any abnormality is seen on X-rays. The knowledge that skeletal metastases are present may significantly alter patient management.

# Assessment of the extent of disease

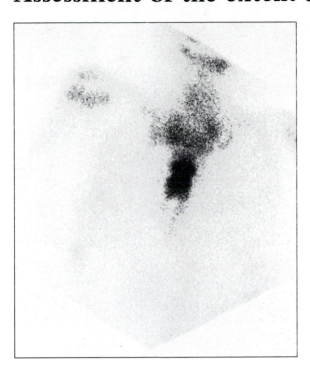

**Figure 4.11**

A patient with carcinoma of the breast who had intensely abnormal radionuclide accumulation throughout the upper half of the sternum. No other abnormality was present in the skeleton. The findings indicated a solitary metastasis involving the sternum and this was confirmed by radiography.

**Figure 4.12**

Carcinoma of the breast.
Bone scan views of skull:
**(a)** anterior, **(b)** left
lateral; **(c)** X–ray of
mandible. There is an
intense focus of increased
tracer uptake in the left
mandible. No other lesion
was present elsewhere in
the skeleton. The X–ray of
the mandible reveals a
lytic lesion, which
corresponds to the
abnormality on the bone
scan. Biopsy revealed a
metastasis from
carcinoma of the breast.

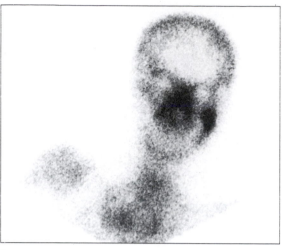

a

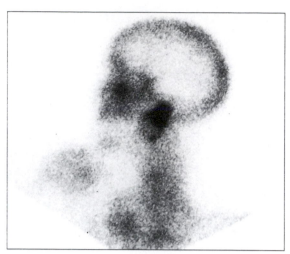

b

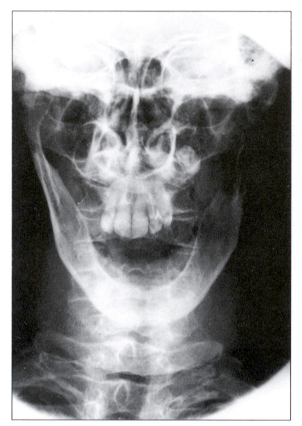

c

## ■ Teaching points

■

While solitary peripheral metastases
are relatively uncommon, they do
occur. There has been some
controversy as to whether routine
views of the skull and lower limbs are
necessary; however, if they are not
obtained, some lesions will be missed.

■

Sites such as the sternum, ribs and
scapula can be difficult to evaluate on
routine radiography, whereas a bone
scan will provide clear visualization of
these areas.

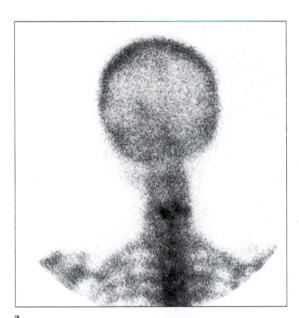

a

**Figure 4.13**

A 72-year-old man with bronchoalveolar cell carcinoma and pain in both shoulders. The posterior view bone scan **(a)** shows a solitary site of increased tracer uptake in the cervical spine. Conventional X-ray examination was normal. The CT scan **(b)** shows vertebral body destruction due to a metastatic tumour.

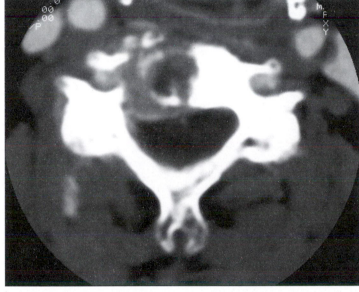

b

**Figure 4.14**

A 50-year-old man with squamous cell lung carcinoma and low back pain due to a metastasis. The posterior view planar bone scan **(a)** shows minimal prominence of activity at L3, which is more convincingly demonstrated and better localized on sagittal **(b)**, coronal **(c)** and transaxial **(d)** SPECT images (arrows). Conventional X-ray examination **(e)** is normal. However, the lesion is obvious on the CT scan **(f)**.

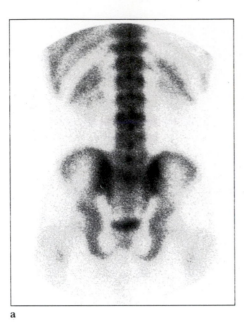

a

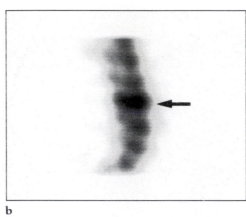

b

c

d

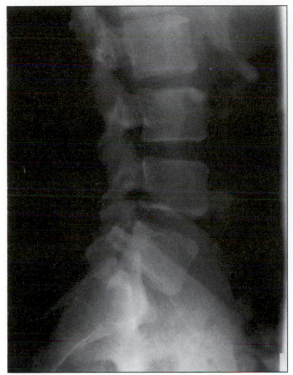

e

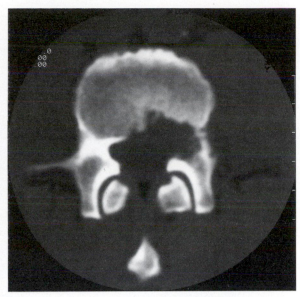

f

**Figure 4.15**

Further examples of patients with carcinoma of the breast who each presented with a single peripheral metastasis. **(a, b)** Solitary skull metastasis; **(c)** solitary metastatic deposit in supraorbital ridge bone; **(d)** solitary metastasis in tibia.

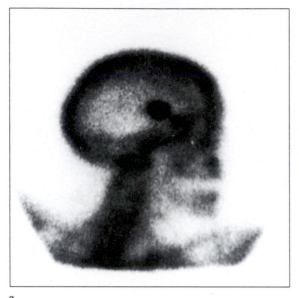

a

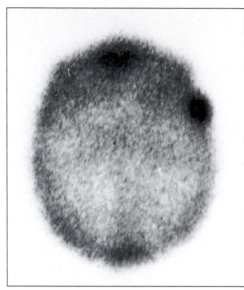

b

c

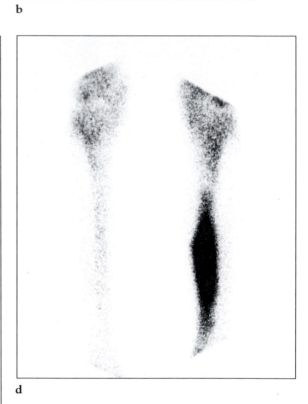

d

# Prediction of fracture

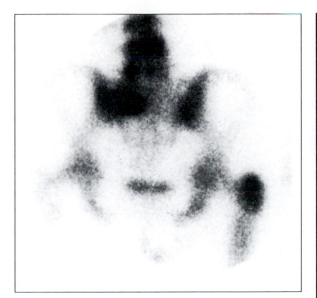

a

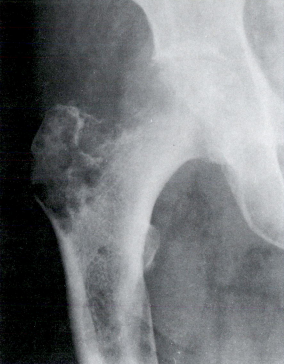

b

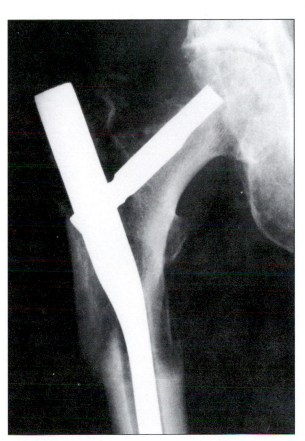

c

**Figure 4.16**

**(a)** Bone scan view, posterior pelvis, upper femora. X-rays: **(b)** right femur and **(c)** following fracture. On the bone scan view there is evidence of metastases involving the lower spine, pelvis, right upper femur and greater trochanter. This patient had extensive metastatic involvement of the skeleton from carcinoma of the breast. The X-ray of the right upper femur shows the presence of metastases, with lytic disease involving the upper right femur and greater trochanter. This patient sustained a pathological fracture, and the X-ray **(c)** shows appearances following surgery.

## ■ Teaching points

■ The bone scan can identify metastases at weight-bearing sites such as the proximal femur, which are at risk of pathological fracture.

■ Given the associated morbidity, the fracture risk should be further evaluated by X-ray and such cases considered for prophylactic internal fixation or radiation therapy.

# Monitoring progress of disease and response to therapy

The bone scan may be used to monitor progression of disease and response to therapy, as reliance on symptoms alone can be misleading. Furthermore, radiographic evidence of healing is slow to manifest, and not possible in the presence of sclerotic metastases.

**Figure 4.17**

Bone scan patterns seen on serial studies.

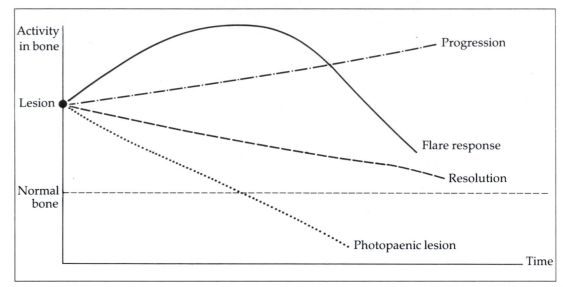

# Progression of disease

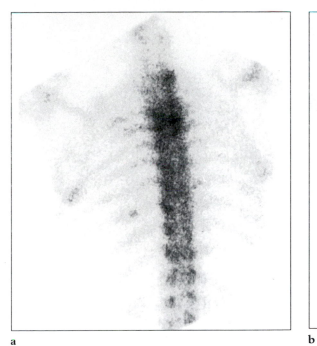

a

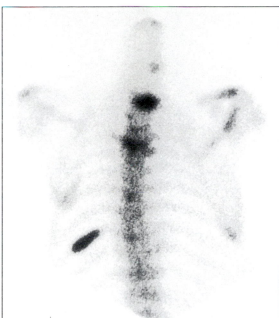

b

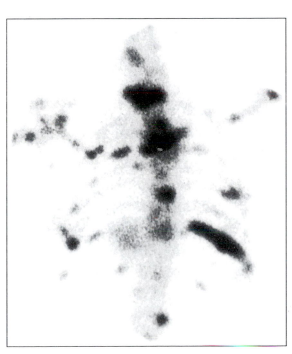

c

**Figure 4.18**

Carcinoma of the prostate. The original bone scan **(a)** shows evidence of metastatic disease in the upper thoracic spine and left 8th rib posteriorly. On subsequent studies obtained 4 months later **(b)** and 8 months later **(c)**, there is clear progression of disease.

**Figure 4.19**

Metastasis at the base of the skull. Bone scan views: **(a)** left lateral skull with corresponding view **(b)** 30 months later. On the second study there is a large focus of increased tracer uptake present at the base of the skull, extending to the left and posteriorly. This patient had carcinoma of the breast, and this lesion represented a solitary metastasis. Having a previously normal study enabled a diagnosis of metastasis to be made with confidence.

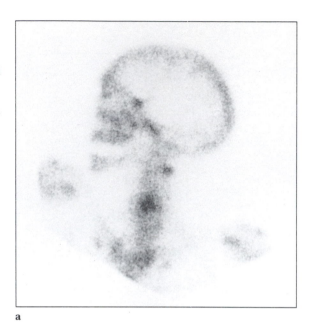
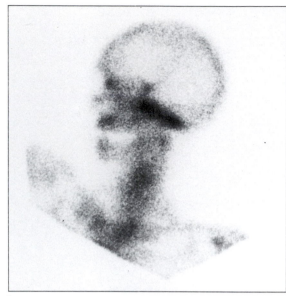

a

b

**Figure 4.20**

Progression of metastases with loss of function in the kidney. On the original study **(a)** of the posterior lumbar spine, there is evidence of metastatic involvement of the skeleton, with some increased uptake of tracer seen in association with the right kidney. On the repeat study **(b)** obtained 3 months later, there has been dramatic progression of disease and the right kidney is no longer visualized. This patient had carcinoma of the prostate, with skeletal metastases. On the original study the right kidney was probably obstructed, with subsequent loss of function.

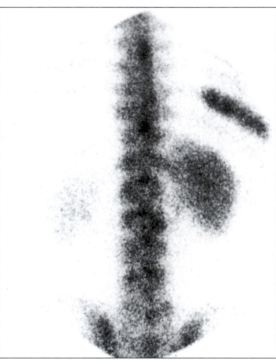
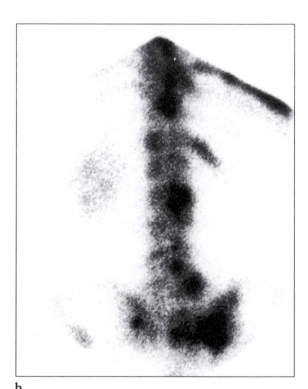

a

b

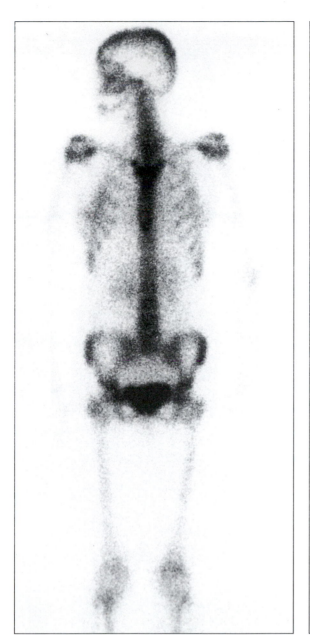

a

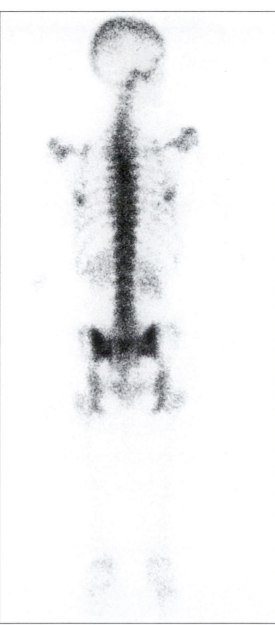

b

**Figure 4.21**

A 37-year-old woman with carcinoma of the breast. The initial bone scan (a, b) is normal. However, the repeat bone scan (c, d) obtained 2 years later shows evidence of metastatic disease, and there is a dramatic progression of disease shown in the subsequent study (e, f) obtained after a further 8 months.

**Figure 4.21** *continued*

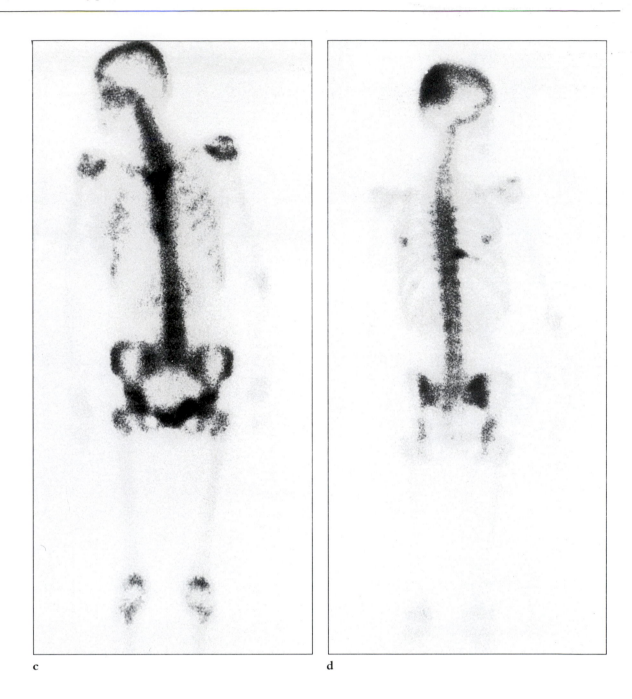

c          d

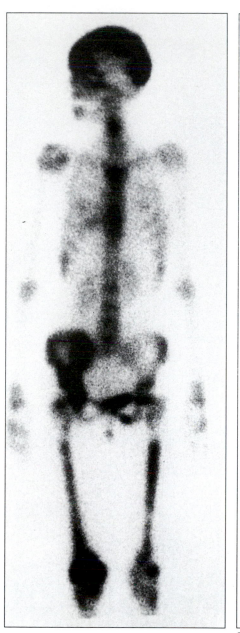

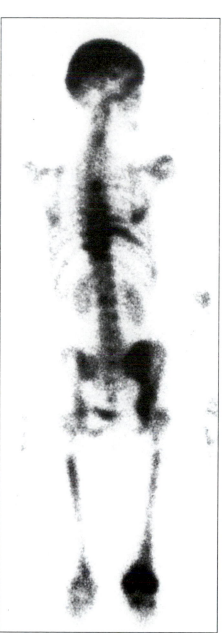

e

f

# Resolution of disease

**Figure 4.22**

A patient with carcinoma of the prostate who had bone scan evidence **(a–c)** of widespread metastatic involvement of the skeleton. However, on the repeat study **(d–f)**, following 10 months treatment with stilboestrol, there has been a dramatic resolution of disease.

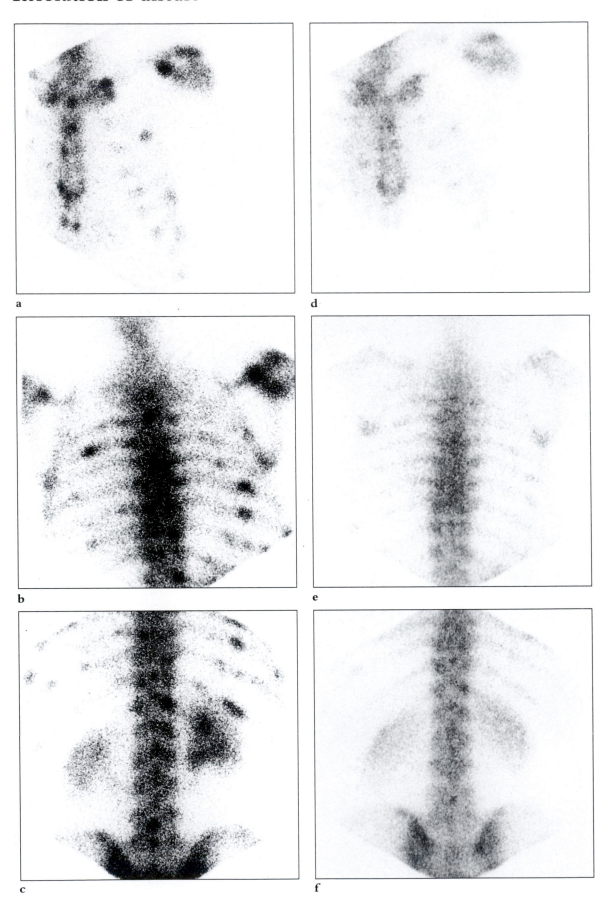

a

d

b

e

c

f

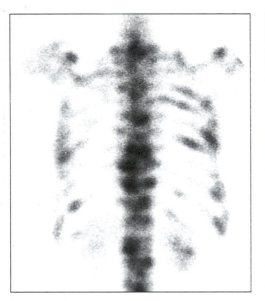

a

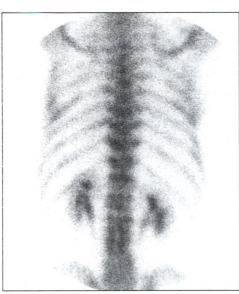

b

**Figure 4.23**

A 70-year-old man with carcinoma of the prostate, who was treated with hormonal therapy and orchiectomy following the demonstration of skeletal metastases on bone scan **(a)**. The follow-up bone scan 1 year later **(b)**, at which time the patient had become asymptomatic, was normal. Two years following orchiectomy, back pain recurred and increased tracer uptake was present in the spine and ribs due to metastases **(c)**.

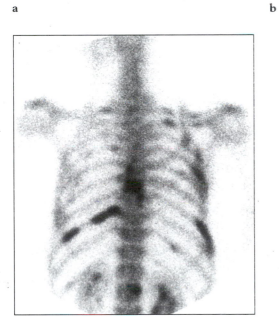

c

**Figure 4.24**

Carcinoma of the breast. The original bone scan **(a, b)** shows evidence of widespread metastatic disease throughout the skeleton. The repeat study **(c, d)** following 3 months chemotherapy, shows a marked improvement in the scan findings.

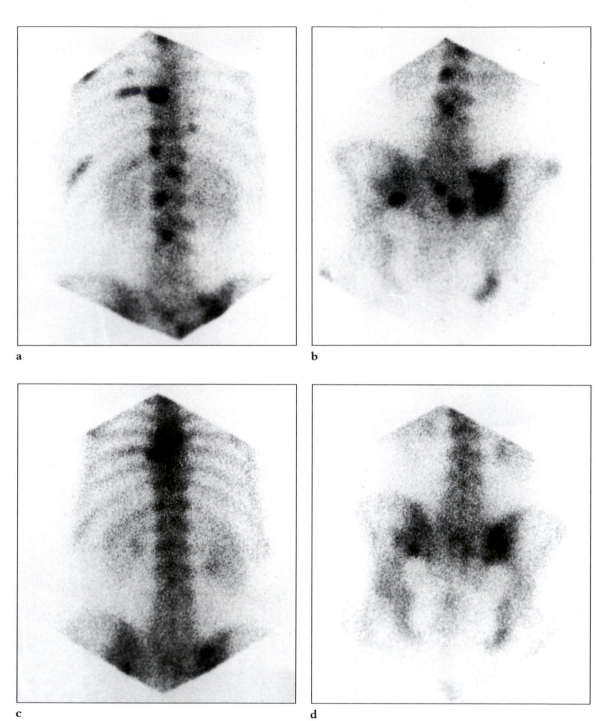

a

b

c

d

# Flare response to therapy

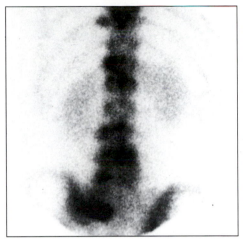

a

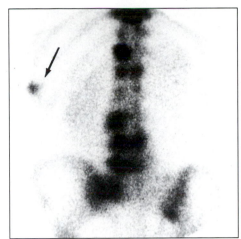

b

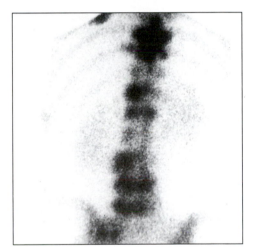

c

**Figure 4.25**

A further case of carcinoma of the breast, in which there was a good response to chemotherapy. The initial scan **(a)** shows widespread metastatic involvement, but the repeat scan **(b)** obtained 3 months later, was thought to show progression of disease as individual lesions appeared more intense and a new focal abnormality was present in the left 10th rib (arrow). However, a subsequent scan **(c)** obtained after a further 3 months shows some evidence of improvement. This is an example of the 'flare' response to therapy, where a scan obtained shortly after instigation of treatment may show an apparent deterioration caused by an intense osteoblastic response reflecting healing. In order to evaluate therapy adequately, there should be a delay of at least 6 months, and perhaps a little longer, between scans.

**Figure 4.26**

Flare reponse with successful therapy.

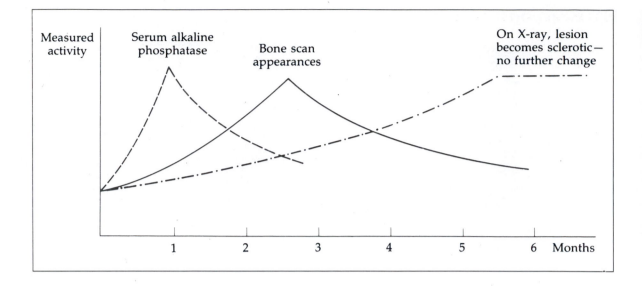

## ■ Teaching point

■ In a patient with metastatic disease, it may not be possible to evaluate response to therapy in the initial months, as apparent deterioration in scan findings may reflect bone healing.

# Radiotherapy

Bone scan appearances in patients who have received radiotherapy are often characteristic.

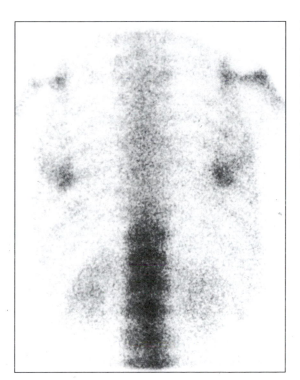

**Figure 4.27**

An example of the characteristic bone scan appearance after radiotherapy. There is generally reduced tracer uptake throughout the thoracic spine, with a sharp cut-off between abnormal and normal bone.

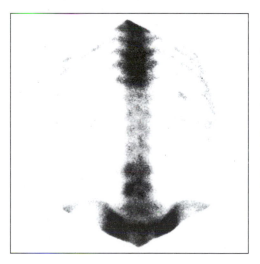

**Figure 4.28**

A patient who received radiotherapy because of severe pain in the lumbar spine. However, there is widespread metastatic disease involving the whole skeleton, and the scan appearances dramatically show the effect of radiotherapy in a patient with a 'superscan' of malignancy.

**Figure 4.29**

A patient with carcinoma of the lung who received radiotherapy for a metastasis in the thoracic spine. Bone scan was requested for reassessment of disease. Marked differential uptake of tracer between the thoracic and lumbar spine is seen, characteristic of previous radiotherapy. However, there is a discrete focus of increased tracer uptake in the left 7th rib posteriorly, which was due to fracture. Appearances are, however, non-specific and X-ray confirmation is necessary.

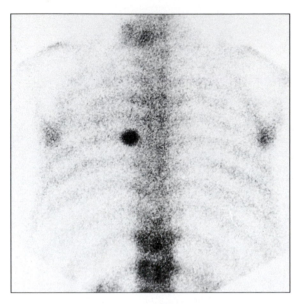

**Figure 4.30**

Fractured ribs following radiotherapy in a patient with carcinoma of the breast. Bone scan view: right anterior chest. There are focal areas of increased tracer uptake in the right 2nd and 3rd ribs anteriorly. X-ray confirmed fractures at these sites. These are pathological fractures secondary to radiation necrosis.

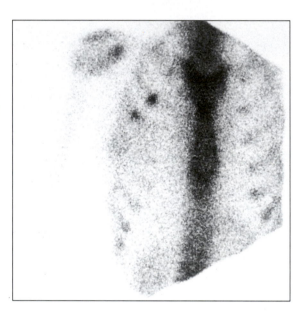

## ■ Teaching point

■
Following radiotherapy, fracture of the ribs may occur spontaneously. This is seen most often in carcinoma of the breast.

# Increased renal uptake of diphosphonate

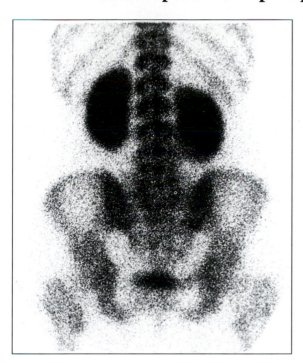

**Figure 4.31**

A patient with carcinoma of the lung being treated with chemotherapy. On the bone scan image, high uptake of tracer is seen in both kidneys. This reflects the renal cytotoxic effect of chemotherapy. However, similar appearances may be seen, on occasion, in patients who are significantly hypercalcaemic.

# Hypertrophic pulmonary osteoarthropathy

## Three cases of hypertrophic pulmonary osteoarthropathy associated with carcinoma of the lung

**Figure 4.32**

On the bone scan images there is diffusely increased tracer uptake, with more focal areas also present, in the cortical aspects of the lower ends of the radius and ulna (a), lower femora (c) and tibiae (d). The X-rays (b, e) confirm a cortical reaction, and the scan findings are typical of hypertrophic pulmonary osteoarthropathy.

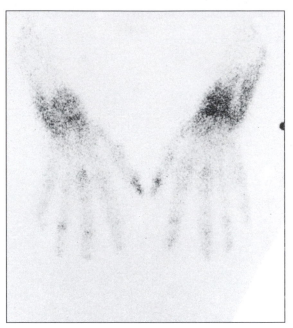

a

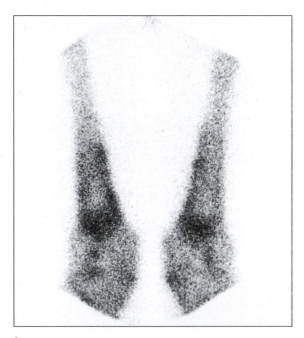

c

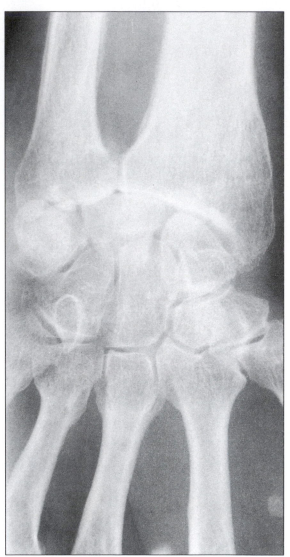

b

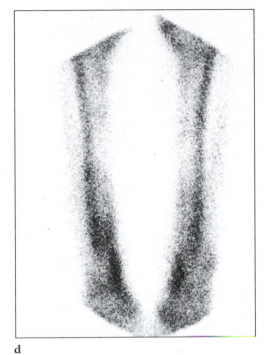

d

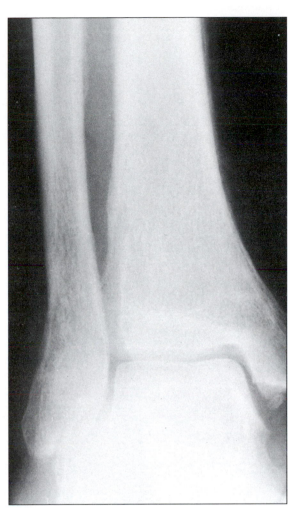

e

**Figure 4.33**

There is increased tracer uptake peripherally in both femoral shafts and the right upper tibia. The scan appearances are typical of a periosteal reaction, and in this case were due to hypertrophic pulmonary osteoarthropathy. Note also that there is increased patellar uptake. This is of no real significance, but has been observed in approximately 50 per cent of cases of hypertrophic pulmonary osteoarthropathy.

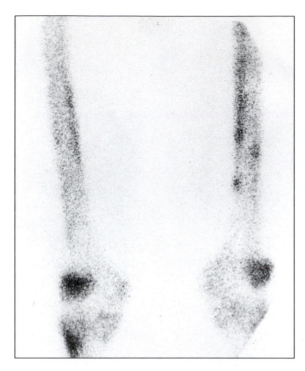

**Figure 4.34**

The bone scan **(a)** shows slight, diffusely increased tracer uptake in the medial aspect of both lower femora, with more focal areas of increased tracer uptake in the left upper femur and lower right femur. The X-ray **(b)** confirms a periosteal reaction at these sites.

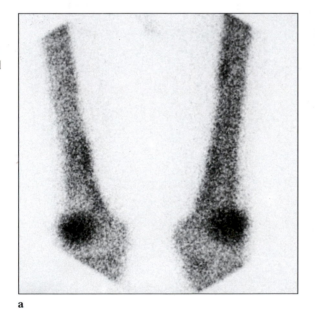

a

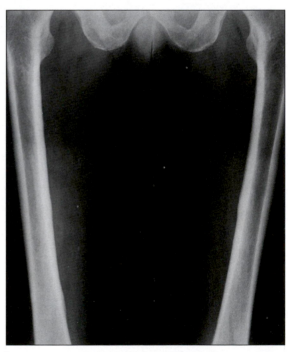

b

# Primary bone tumours

## Table 4.1 Classification of malignant primary bone tumours

| Site of origin | Tumour |
| --- | --- |
| Skeletal connective tissues | Osteogenic sarcoma |
| | Chondrosarcoma |
| | Fibrosarcoma |
| | Giant-cell tumour |
| Other skeletal components | Liposarcoma |
| Unknown | Ewings' tumour |

## Ewing's tumour

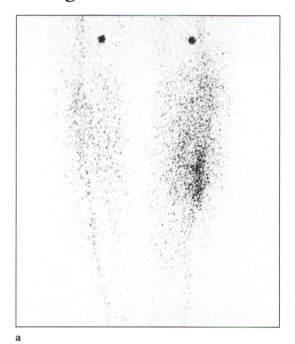

a

b

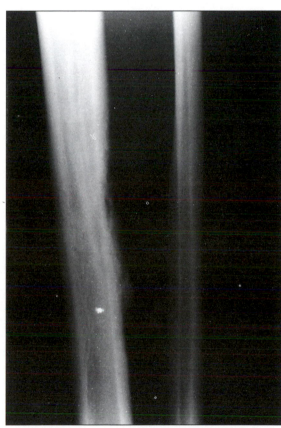

c

**Figure 4.35**

A 20-year-old woman with Ewing's tumour. Bone scan views of anterior tibiae: **(a)** dynamic and **(b)** static. There is increased vascularity and increased tracer uptake at the left mid-tibia. The tumour is shown on the X-ray **(c)**.

**Figure 4.36**

A 29-year-old man with Ewing's tumour involving the right upper humerus. Bone scan views: **(a)** anterior chest and **(b)** post-surgery. On the original study there is markedly increased tracer uptake involving the right upper humerus at the site of a known Ewing's tumour. On the repeat study following surgery, a right humeral prosthesis can be seen. In addition, there is some increased tracer uptake associated with the right coracoid, which presumably related to surgical intervention.

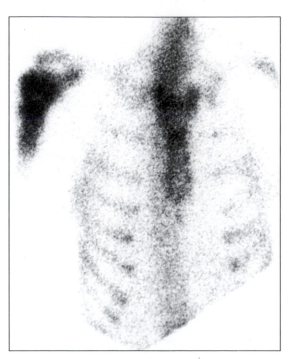

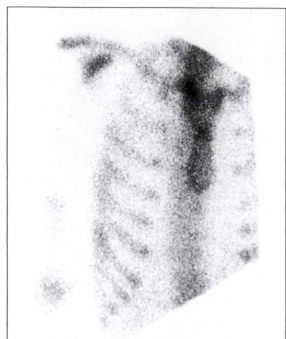

a

b

**Figure 4.37**

Bone scan showing massively increased tracer uptake in the right lower humerus caused by a Ewing's tumour.

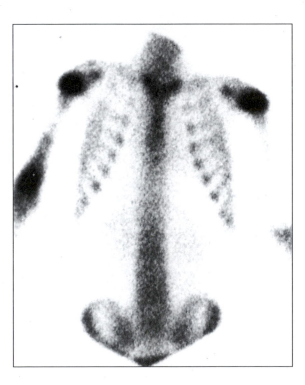

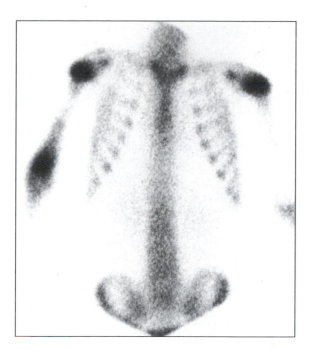

**Figure 4.38**

Bone scan findings , similar to those in Figure 4.37, but in this case the diagnosis was subsequently found to be acute lymphatic leukaemia. The scan appearances in isolation are most likely to be due to a primary bone tumour, rather than leukaemic infiltration.

# ■ Teaching point

■

Although the bone scan is sensitive for lesion detection, scan appearances are non-specific.

# Osteogenic sarcoma

**Figure 4.39**

Osteogenic sarcoma of the right upper tibia. Bone scan views: **(a)** anterior, and **(b)** posterior. There is no evidence of metastatic disease elsewhere in the skeleton. Skeletal metastases are relatively uncommon at the time of presentation with osteogenic sarcoma and occur more frequently with Ewing's tumour.

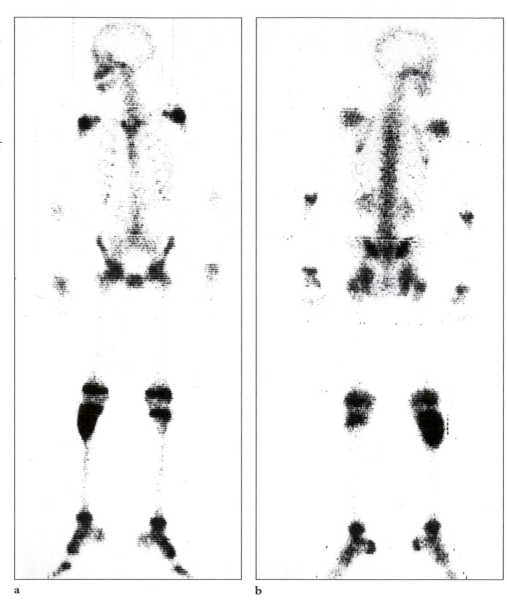

a                                     b

**Figure 4.40**

Osteogenic sarcoma with massive abnormal tracer accumulation in lung metastases. It is well recognized that pulmonary deposits may take up $^{99m}$Tc-MDP.

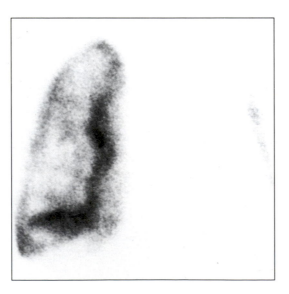

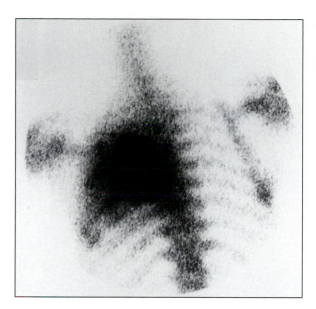

**Figure 4.41**

A further case of osteogenic sarcoma, with massive abnormal tracer accumulation throughout the left lung caused by pulmonary and pleural deposits.

**Figure 4.42**

An unusual case of osteogenic sarcoma in a 28-year-old woman. Bone scan views of the upper thorax: **(a)** anterior; **(b)** posterior; **(c)** CT scan. The bone scan images show massive focal tracer accumulation in the region of the cervical spine, extending out to the left. The CT scan confirms a destructive lesion involving the cervical spine and extending into soft tissue. This was subsequently shown to be an osteogenic sarcoma.

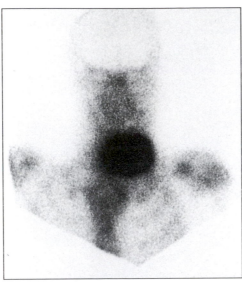

a

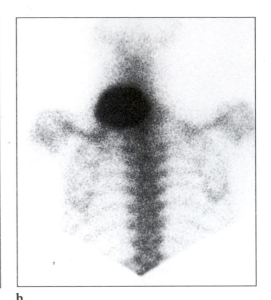

b

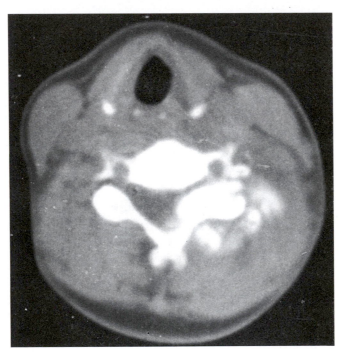

c

# Chondrosarcoma

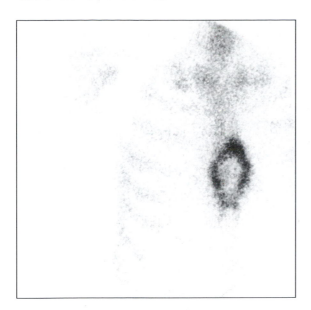

**Figure 4.43**

An elderly man who presented with a sternal mass. The bone scan image of the anterior chest shows increased tracer uptake in the sternum, particularly at the peripheral borders, with a relative photon-deficient area at its centre. Biopsy of the sternal mass revealed chondrosarcoma.

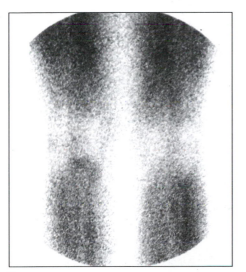

a

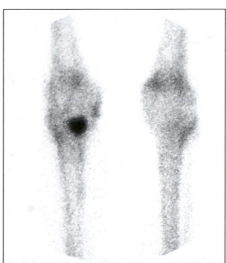

b

**Figure 4.44**

A 40-year-old woman with right knee pain and no history of trauma. The blood pool image **(a)** shows a slight increase in vascularity at a site where there is intense tracer uptake on the bone scan **(b)**. Conventional X-ray examination **(c)** shows calcifications suggestive of a chondroma or chondrosarcoma. The CT scan **(d)** shows bone destruction in addition to the calcifications. Biopsy established the diagnosis of a low-grade chondrosarcoma.

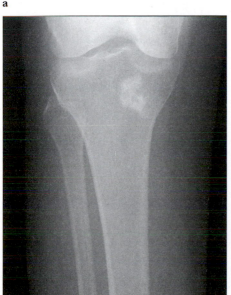

c

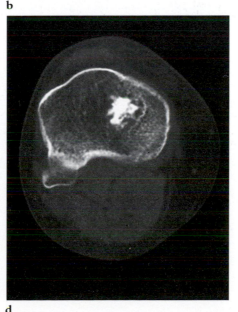

d

## Giant cell tumour

**Figure 4.45**

A 13-year-old girl treated surgically for giant cell tumour of C2. The posterior view bone scan **(a)** before surgery shows a solitary site of increased tracer uptake at C2. The CT scan **(b)** demonstrates a lytic lesion at this site.

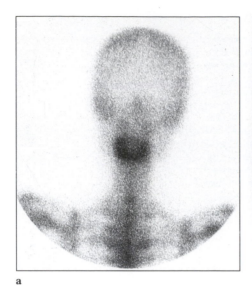

a

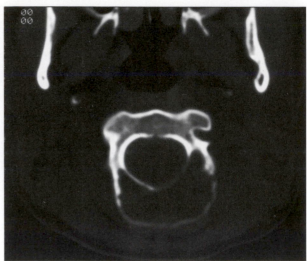

b

## ■ Teaching point

■

Giant cell tumours have varying malignant potential.

# Primary lymphoma of bone

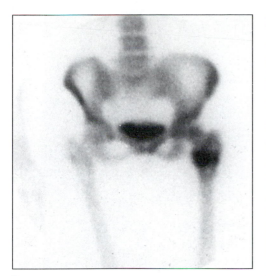

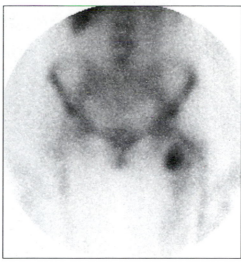

a

c

**Figure 4.46**

A 31-year-old woman who presented with left hip pain. The bone scan of the anterior pelvis **(a)** shows increased tracer uptake corresponding to the destructive lesion noted on X-ray **(b)**. The $^{67}$Ga image **(c)** also shows increased tracer uptake by the lesion, which was subsequently shown to be a primary lymphoma of bone.

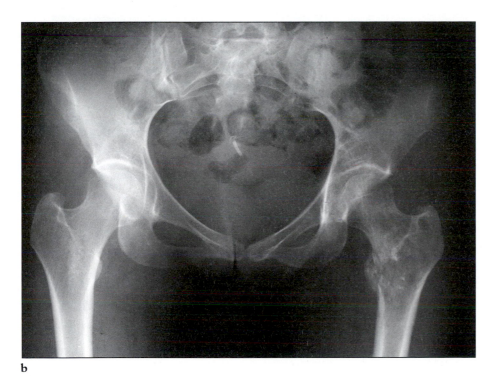

b

# Eosinophilic granuloma

**Figure 4.47**

A 10-year-old boy with right arm pain. The bone scan of the right arm **(a)** shows increased uptake in the distal humerus. The X-ray **(b)** shows a permeative destructive process at this site. Biopsy eventually established the diagnosis of eosinophilic granuloma.

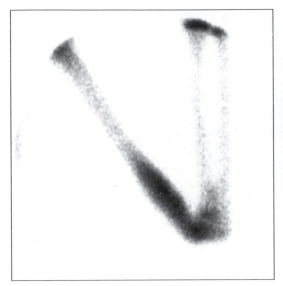

a

b

# Clinical indication for bone scanning: investigation of benign bone disease

**5**

- Orthopaedic disorders
- Fractures
- Sports injuries
- Benign bone tumours
- Infection
- Arthritis
- Metabolic bone disease and other osteopathies
- Paget's disease
- Metabolic activity of a lesion

## Orthopaedic disorders

### Evaluation of hip prosthesis

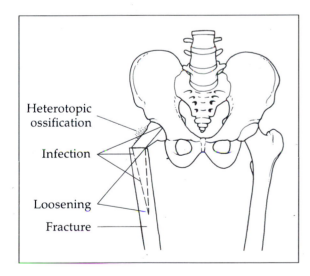

**Figure 5.1**

The painful prosthesis.

Heterotopic ossification

Infection

Loosening

Fracture

**Figure 5.2**

Loosening. Bone scan views of anterior right hip and upper femur: **(a)** original study and **(b)** 1 year later. On the original study, the scan appearances 1 year after insertion of a right hip prosthesis are normal. However, 1 year later, the patient complained of recurrence of pain in the right hip and the repeat scan shows a focus of increased activity at the tip of the prosthesis (arrow). The scan findings are typical of loosening of a prosthesis.

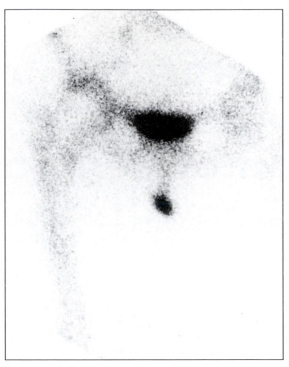

a

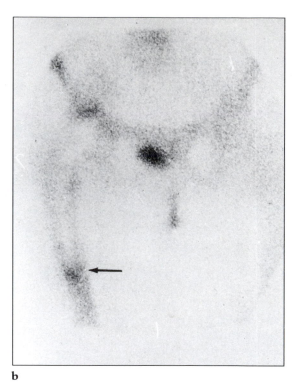

b

**Figure 5.3**

A 63-year-old woman with bilateral hip prostheses. Bone scan view of the anterior femora. There is loosening of the left hip prosthesis. Note the intense focus of increased uptake at the tip of the femoral component which is displaced medially.

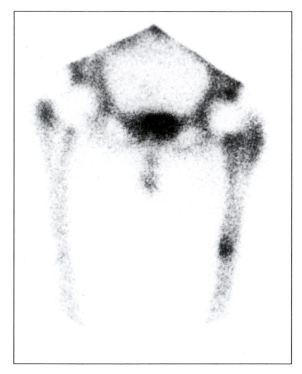

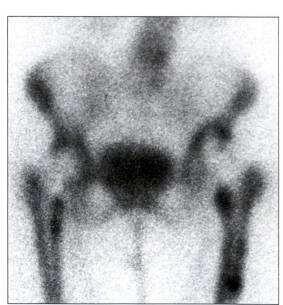

**Figure 5.4**

An infected and loose left total hip prosthesis in a 60-year-old woman: bone scan view of the anterior femora. Bilateral hip prostheses were inserted 2 years previously. There is significantly increased uptake at the bony margins adjacent to both the femoral and acetabular components of the left hip prosthesis.

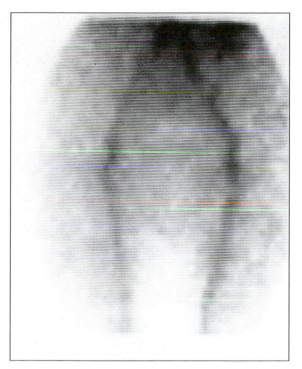

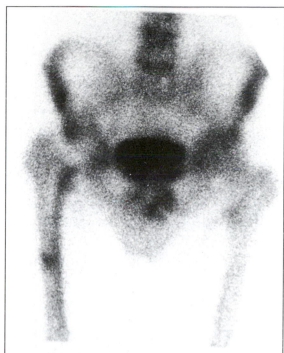

a

b

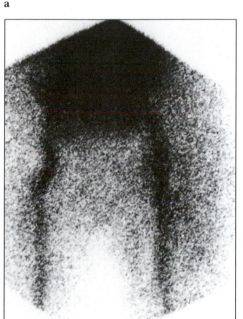

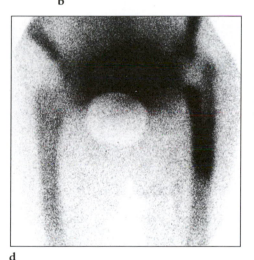

c

d

**Figure 5.5**

Differentiation between loosening of prosthesis and infection.

*Case 1:* Loosening. There is a discrete focus of increased tracer uptake at the tip of the femoral prosthesis **(b)**. The blood pool image **(a)** is normal.

*Case 2:* Infected prosthesis. There is markedly increased tracer uptake associated with the femoral component of the prosthesis **(d)**. The blood pool image **(c)** indicates increased vascularity at that site.

## ■ Teaching point

■

The time interval following surgery is important. Persistent abnormality on the bone scan may be seen for up to a year after surgery, and even longer in the region of the greater trochanter when this area has sustained significant trauma. In some cases it will not be possible to differentiate between infection and loosening on the basis of the bone scan alone, and a repeat study with either gallium or indium-labelled white cells should provide additional information.

**Figure 5.6**

A 60-year-old man who complained of continued severe right hip pain 1 month following total hip replacement. The blood pool image **(a)** shows a slight increase in vascularity over the acetabular prosthetic component and the joint space. Bone scan images **(b, c)** show increased tracer uptake about all bony margins adjacent to prosthetic components, which is to be expected with active continuing repair and remodelling 1 month following orthopaedic surgery. The $^{67}$Ga image **(d)** shows moderately intense abnormal activity over the acetabulum and the joint space. The abnormal $^{67}$Ga activity extends well beyond the boundary of the increased $^{99m}$Tc-MDP uptake, a combination of findings which is suspicious for infection. Hip aspiration confirmed the diagnosis of septic arthritis.

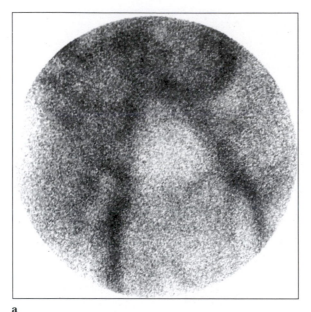

a

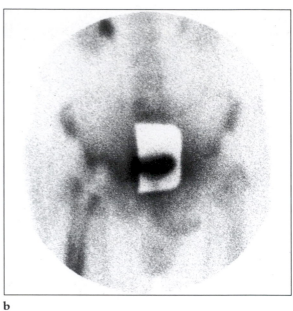

b

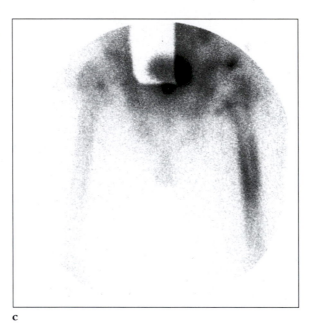

c

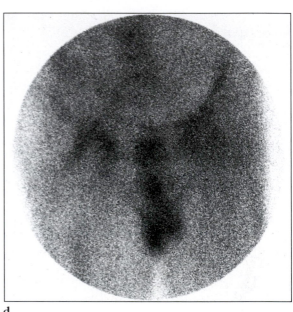

d

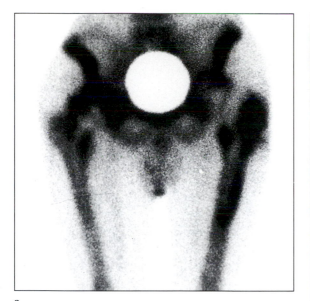

a

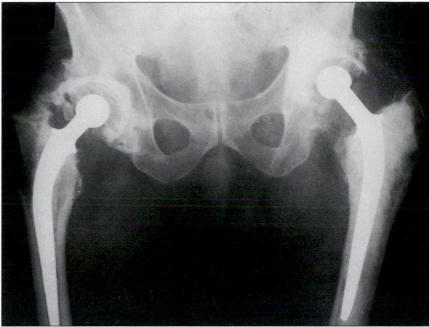

b

**Figure 5.7**

Heterotopic ossification. Bilateral hip prostheses are present. The bone scan (a) shows increased uptake of tracer on the right, in the region of the femoral neck, bridging the acetabulum and greater trochanter. These appearances are typical of heterotopic ossification, which is confirmed on the X-ray (b). The scan findings on the left are quite abnormal, with markedly increased tracer uptake in the region of the left greater trochanter and along the lateral border of the femoral component of the prosthesis. Infection cannot be excluded.

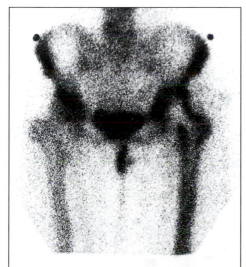

a

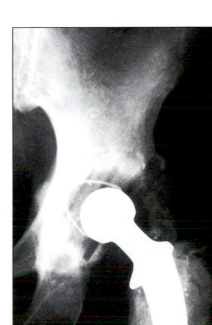

b

**Figure 5.8 (a, b)**

A further case of heterotopic ossification associated with a left femoral prosthesis.

# Plantar fasciitis

**Figure 5.9**

A 44-year-old man who complained of 3 months of persistent right heel pain. There was no history of trauma. The plantar view blood pool image **(a)** shows increased vascularity over the plantar surface of the right heel. Both plantar **(b)** and right lateral **(c)** bone scans show increased tracer uptake along the plantar surface of the right calcaneus at the site of attachment of the plantar aponeurosis. The findings are typical of plantar fasciitis.

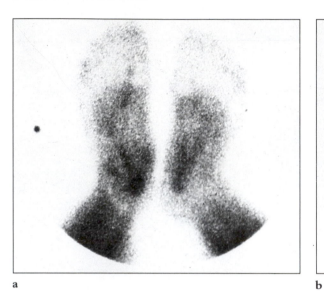

a

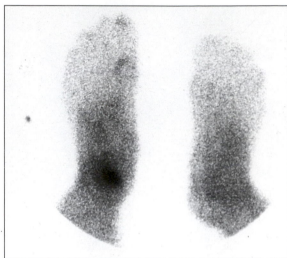

b

c

# Calcaneal stress fracture

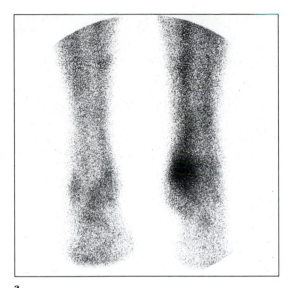

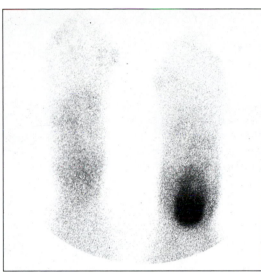

**Figure 5.10**

A 57-year-old man who complained of left heel pain, which began shortly after he underwent total hip replacement and resumed walking. The anterior blood pool image **(a)** shows increased vascularity to the left ankle and heel. Plantar **(b)** and left lateral **(c)** bone scan images show intense tracer uptake extending deep into the neck of the calcaneus. Subsequent X-ray examination showed findings typical of a stress fracture.

a

b

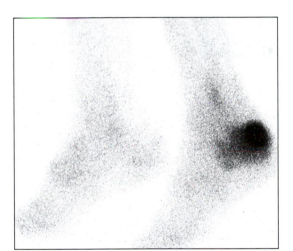

c

## Os trigonum syndrome

**Figure 5.11**

A 35-year-old woman with right heel pain. The X-ray **(a)** shows an os trigonum, an accessory ossicle posterior to the talus. The lateral bone scan image **(b)** shows increased tracer uptake in the os trigonum, an abnormal finding suggesting that this is the site of the patient's heel pain. Pain was relieved following resection of the os trigonum.

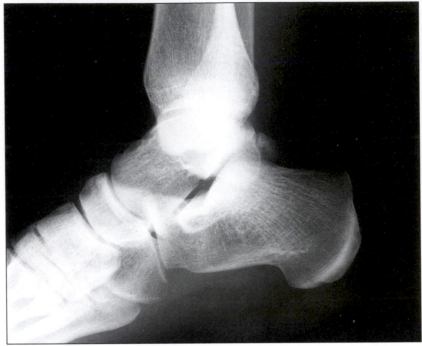

a

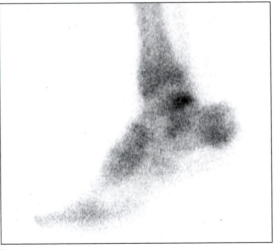

b

## Frostbite

**Figure 5.12**

Frostbite injuries sustained by a shoeless 45-year-old man who slept outside in cold weather. A medial view of the right foot shows absent tracer uptake distally in the toes and throughout much of the calcaneus. Tissue necrosis eventually developed.

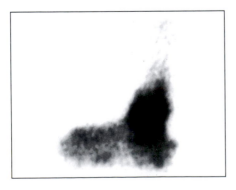

# Avascular necrosis

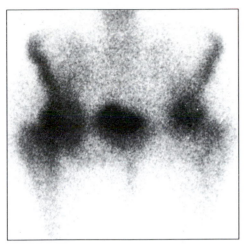

a

**Figure 5.13**

**(a)** Bone scan view of anterior pelvis and hips; **(b)** X-ray of pelvis. This patient was taking steroid therapy for nephrotic syndrome. The bone scan shows intensely increased tracer uptake in the region of both hips. The scan findings are compatible with avascular necrosis, which is confirmed on the X-ray.

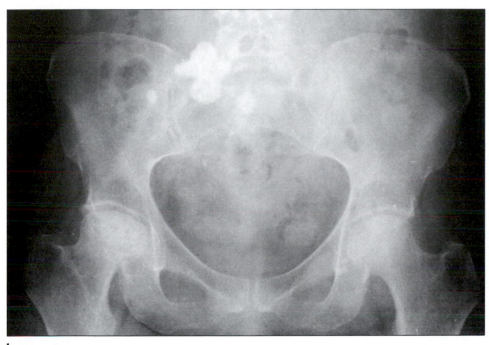

b

**Figure 5.14**

A 30-year-old man who was receiving steroids for hepatitis. Bone scan views: **(a)** pelvis, **(b)** femur; **(c, d)** X-rays of upper and lower femur. It is apparent that there is strikingly increased tracer uptake in the region of the right femoral head **(a)**, which corresponds to the avascular necrosis and dislocation seen on the X-ray **(c)**. There is also diffusely increased tracer uptake throughout the shaft of the right femur, with focal increased uptake at the lower femur **(b)**. The X-ray **(d)** shows a fracture at that site. The more general increased uptake throughout the shaft of the right femur is due to disuse osteoporosis.

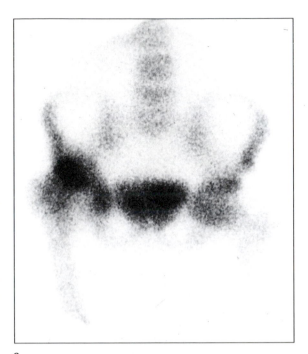

a

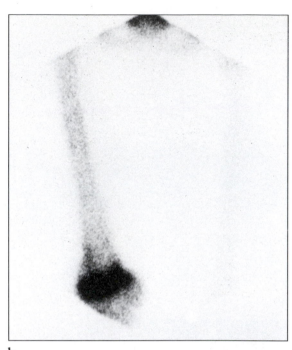

b

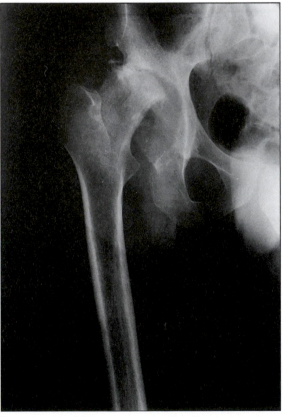

c

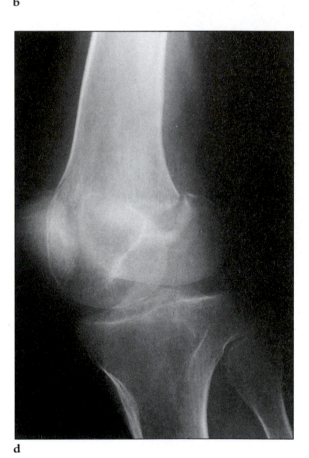

d

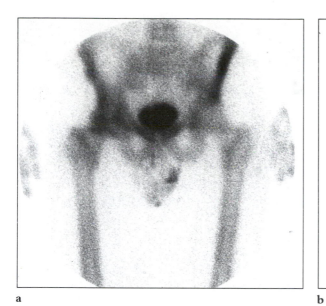

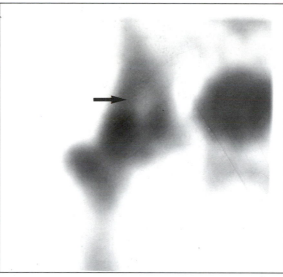

a

b

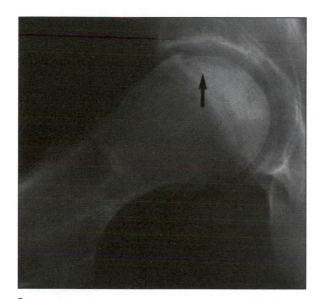

c

**Figure 5.15**

A 45-year-old woman with no predisposing risk factors for avascular necrosis who complained of right hip pain. Anterior planar (a) and coronal plane SPECT (b) images should be examined for evidence of decreased tracer uptake within the femoral head, which is typical of avascular necrosis. A zone of relatively decreased activity within the right femoral head is better seen on the SPECT image (arrow). Sclerosis and cortical disruption of the right femoral head on X-ray (c) also suggest avascular necrosis (arrow).

**Figure 5.16**

A 58-year-old man with avascular necrosis of the left femoral head following radiation therapy. Both planar **(a)** and coronal plane SPECT **(b)** bone scans show a zone of relatively decreased activity medially in the left femoral head, with surrounding regions of increased tracer uptake.

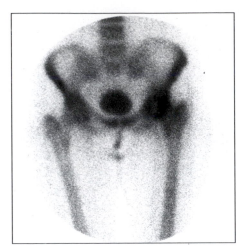

a

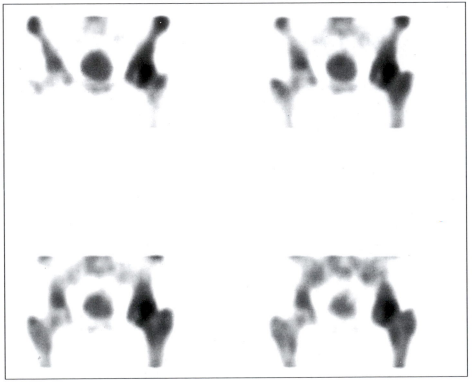

b

## ■ Teaching point

■ High resolution collimation is often needed in order to visualize a photon-deficient avascular lesion within the femoral head. The photon-deficient defect typical of AVN is seen even more frequently when SPECT bone scans are obtained.

# Problems in identifying avascular necrosis on SPECT images

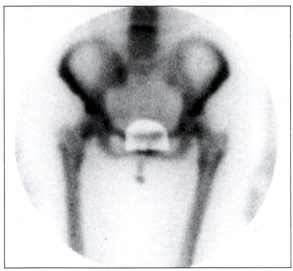

a

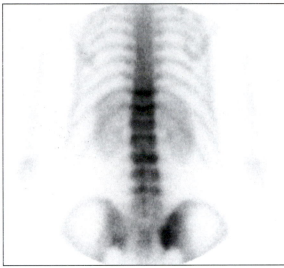

b

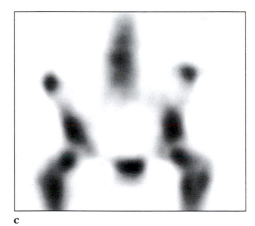

c

**Figure 5.17**

A 40-year-old osteoporotic liver transplant patient who was being treated with steroids and who complained of back, pelvis and hip pain. Bone scan views: **(a)** anterior pelvis, **(b)** posterior thoracolumbar spine, and **(c)** coronal plane SPECT image through the femoral necks. Increased tracer uptake in the spine and right sacroiliac joint is due to known fractures. Increased activity along the medial cortical margins of both femoral necks on the planar image has an appearance typical for stress fractures. The appearance of these femoral neck stress fractures on the SPECT image mimics the relatively decreased femoral head activity seen with avascular necrosis. X-rays of hips were normal.

**Figure 5.18**

Adolescent growth plate activity also may mimic avascular necrosis. For this 17-year-old man, normally prominent growth plate activity is present adjacent to the femoral heads on both planar **(a)** and SPECT **(b)** images.

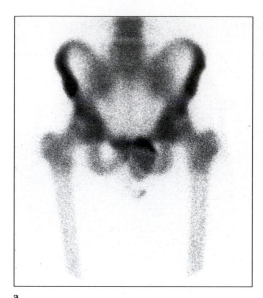

a

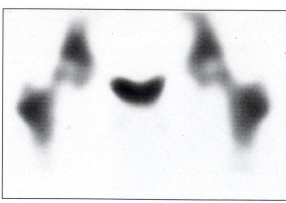

b

a

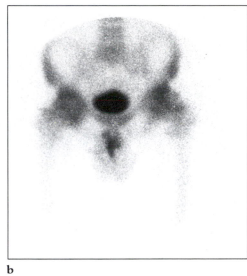

b

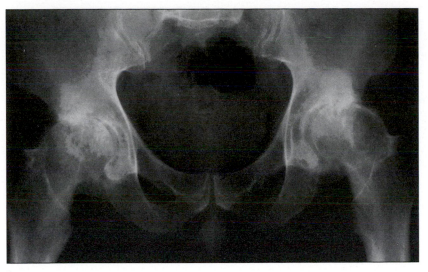

c

**Figure 5.19**

Advanced osteoarthritis also may mimic avascular necrosis, due predominantly to increased tracer uptake associated with osteophyte formation. This is a 75-year-old man with advanced osteo-arthritis of the hips, as shown on the X-ray **(a)**. The anterior view planar **(b)** and serial anterior-to-posterior coronal plane SPECT images **(c)** reflect these radiographic findings. If interpreted without radiographic correlation, the bone scans might be confused with avascular necrosis of the femoral heads.

## ■ Teaching point

■ The SPECT bone scan appearances of growth plates, osteoarthritis or femoral neck stress fractures can mimic the photon-deficient area typical of femoral head avascular necrosis as illustrated in the above three cases.

**Figure 5.20**

A 41-year-old man who presented with right hip pain. A photon-deficient area in the right femoral head with adjacent zones of increased tracer uptake typical of avascular necrosis is well seen on the planar **(a)** but not the coronal SPECT **(b)** images. The failure of SPECT to detect the photon-deficient area may be explained by the bladder-filling artefact, which in part obscures the right femoral head (see Figure 2.53).

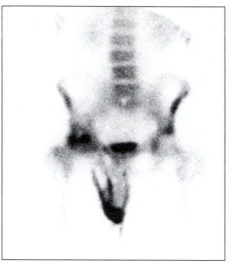

a

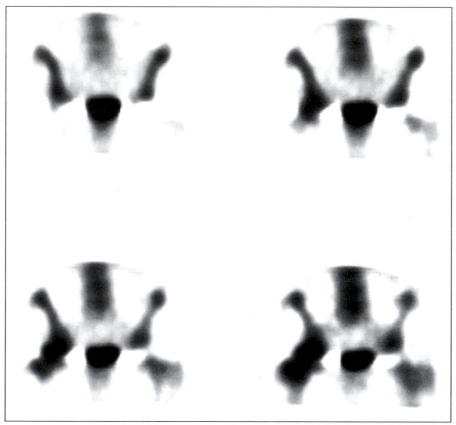

b

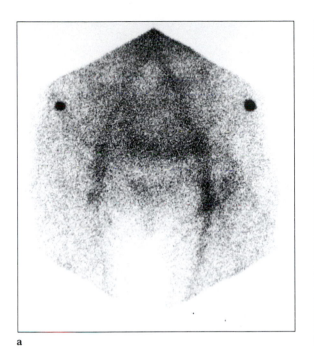

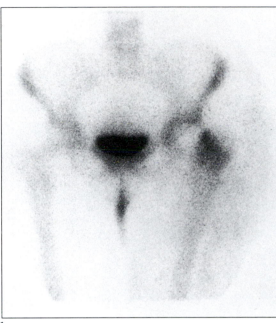

a                                              b

**Figure 5.21**

Avascular necrosis following fracture. Bone scan views of anterior pelvis and femora: **(a)** blood pool and **(b)** delayed image. This patient sustained a subcapital fracture of the left femur, which was fixed with compression screws. The blood pool image shows reduced vascularity to the left femoral head. On the delayed image, there is an obvious photon-deficient area in the region of the left femoral head, together with some increased tracer uptake at the greater trochanter, which presumably reflects surgical intervention. The scan appearances indicate that the left femoral head is no longer viable.

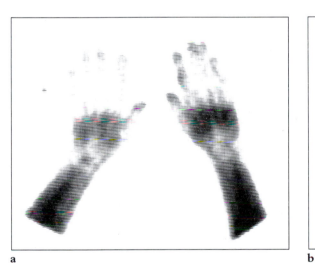

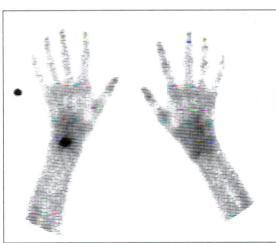

a                                              b

**Figure 5.22**

Avascular necrosis of the carpal lunate (Kienböck's) in a patient who complained of pain in the right hand. Bone scan views of hands: **(a)** blood pool and **(b)** delayed image. X-rays suggested avascular necrosis of the lunate bone. The bone scan confirms a discrete focus of increased tracer uptake associated with the lunate. There is also increased blood flow to that site.

**Figure 5.23**

Perthes disease. Bone scan views: **(a)** normal study; **(b)** blood pool and **(c)** static views of anterior pelvis and femora in a 14-year-old boy with Perthes disease. Although the resolution is poor on the blood pool study, there is probably reduced blood flow in the region of the left femoral head. On the delayed images, there is a clear photon-deficient area in the femoral epiphysis on the left.

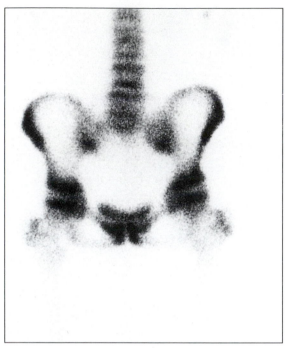

a

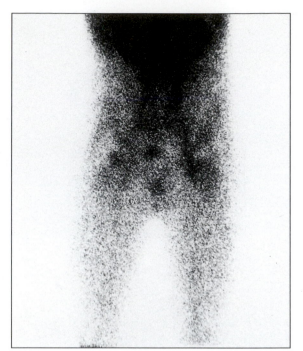

b

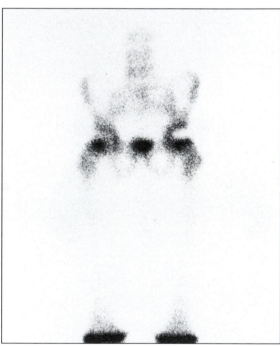

c

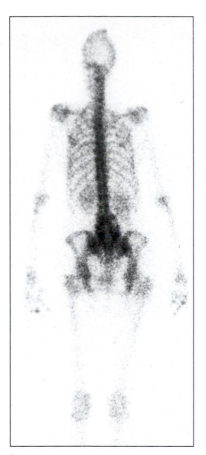

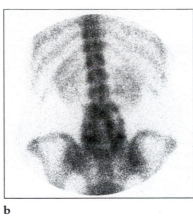

a

b

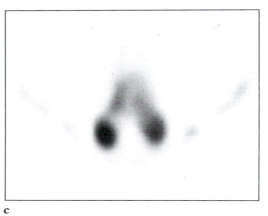

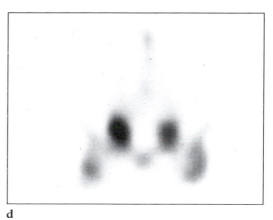

c

d

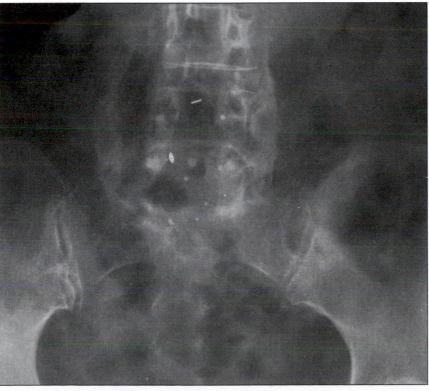

e

**Figure 5.24**

Pseudoarthrosis. Bone scan images: **(a)** whole body posterior view; **(b)** high resolution collimator view of the posterior lumbar spine; **(c)** SPECT transaxial and **(d)** coronal views; together with X-ray **(e)** in a woman patient, 3 years following spinal fusion and 1 year following repeat surgical exploration for persistent severe low back pain. While not evident on the total body image, the planar study shows focal increased uptake over the lower end of both sides of the bony fusion mass. Both the site of this abnormality and the marked intensity of tracer uptake are better appreciated on the SPECT images. Surgical exploration identified pseudoarthroses, and pain was relieved following the repeat fusion.

**Figure 5.25**

A 60-year-old woman who complained of persistent low back pain more than 1 year following a lower-lumbar spinal fusion. The X-ray **(a)** shows both advanced osteoarthritic changes about the L4–L5 intervertebral disc space and possible pseudoarthrosis within the fusion mass. Increased tracer uptake at this level is evident on posterior **(b)** and posterior oblique **(c, d)** bone scan images. However, a mid-line sagittal SPECT image **(e)** along with coronal SPECT image **(f)** through the middle of the bony fusion mass were needed to localize the most intense tracer uptake to the vertebral body end plates rather than the fusion mass.

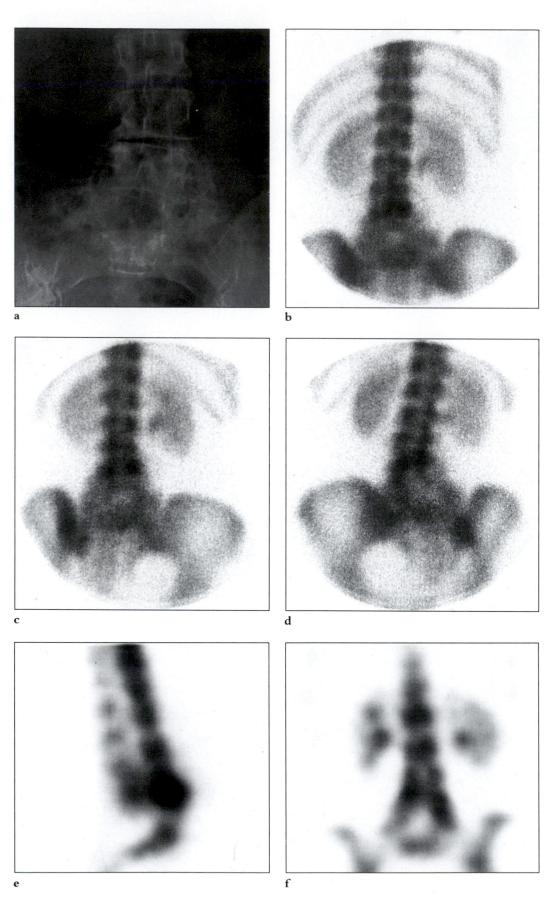

a

b

c

d

e

f

# Differentiation between avascular necrosis and osteoarthritis of the knee

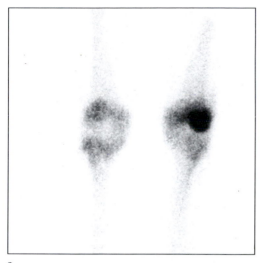

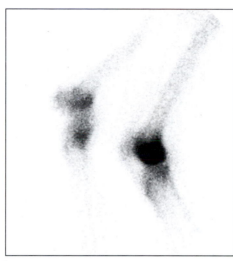

a                                                   b

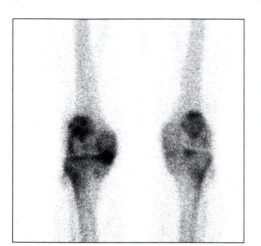

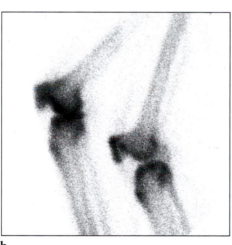

a                                                   b

**Figure 5.26**
A 35-year-old woman, treated with steroids, who complained of left knee pain. Anterior (a) and lateral (b) bone scans show intense tracer uptake extending from the subchondral bone of the lateral femoral condyle deep into the metaphysis. The X-ray showed changes consistent with avascular necrosis.

**Figure 5.27**
A 60-year-old woman with recent worsening of right knee pain and clinical suspicion of avascular necrosis of the lateral femoral condyle. The anterior (a) and lateral (b) bone scan views show increased tracer uptake in the subchondral bone adjacent to the medial and lateral compartments of the painful right knee, along with increased patellar uptake. The more intense medial compartment uptake is often seen with osteoarthritis. Without extension of increased tracer uptake into the metaphysis of the femoral condyles, there is no evidence of avascular necrosis.

## ■ Teaching point

■ The location rather than the intensity of increased tracer uptake makes it possible to distinguish osteoarthritis from avascular necrosis. In osteoarthritis, increased tracer uptake is confined to the subchondral bone adjacent to the articular surfaces, with both the femoral condyle and the tibial plateau often involved. In avascular necrosis of the femoral condyle, increased tracer uptake extends from the joint surface deep into the metaphysis. Avascular necrosis of the tibial plateau is rare but does occur.

# Fractures

## Fractured ribs

**Figure 5.28**

An elderly woman who had suffered a fall. Bone scan views of posterior thoracic spine: **(a)** original study and **(b)** 11 months later. On the original bone scan, multiple focal abnormalities are present in a linear pattern in the right posterior ribs. The scan appearances are diagnostic of fracture. On the repeat study, there is almost complete resolution, indicating healing of the fractures.

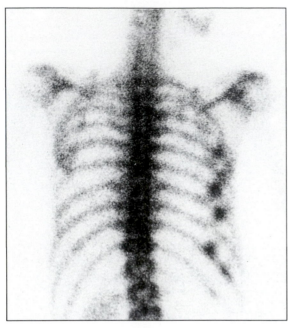

a

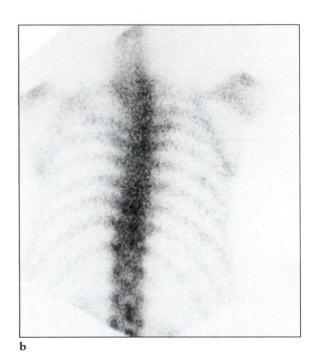

b

**Figure 5.29**

A 50-year-old man who was involved in an automobile accident: bone scan view of the anterior chest. Note that there are multiple focal abnormalities bilaterally in the ribs, in a linear pattern. Focal abnormalities are also present in the upper and lower sternum. The abnormalities are due to multiple fractures following trauma. This pattern of abnormalities often occurs in an automobile accident in which the victim's chest hits the steering wheel.

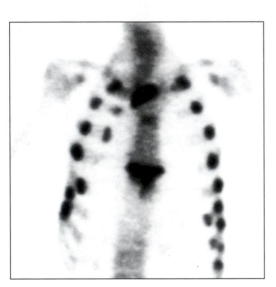

# Fractures of the sacrum

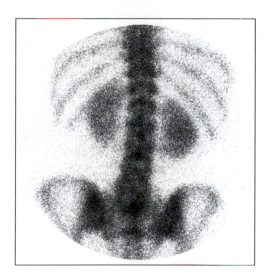

**Figure 5.30**

A 51-year-old woman who had been asymptomatic following a lumbar laminectomy now complained of recurrent low back pain. The bone scan shows a thin linear band of increased activity running transversely across the mid-sacrum, just below the level of the sacroiliac joints. Even though X-ray studies were normal, the bone scan was interpreted as typical of a transverse fracture of the mid-sacrum. On further questioning, the patient recalled that the pain began after a fall. Six months later the patient was asymptomatic.

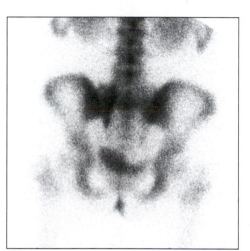

a

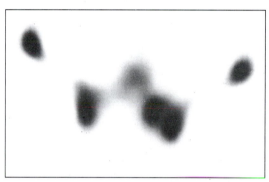

b

**Figure 5.31**

A 27-year-old woman who suffered a sacral fracture. The site of injury is well demonstrated on a posterior planar bone scan **(a)**, a transaxial SPECT bone scan through the mid-sacrum **(b)** and a coronal CT scan **(c)**.

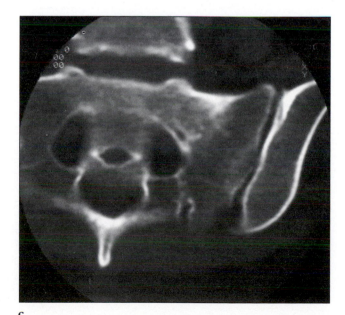

c

**Figure 5.32**

A 60-year-old woman who complained of continued right hip pain 1 week after a fall. X-rays of the hip and pelvis were normal. To exclude the possibility of a non-displaced femoral neck fracture, a bone scan was performed. Anterior (a) and RAO (b) bone scan views show increased tracer uptake in the right-sided superior and inferior pubic rami, along with the right sacroiliac joint. This combination of findings is typical of a pelvic ring fracture due to lateral compression or vertical shear. The RAO view shows that the acetabulum is not involved.

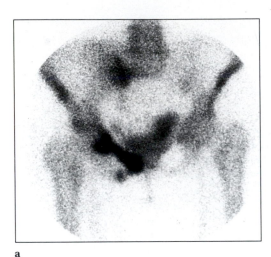

a

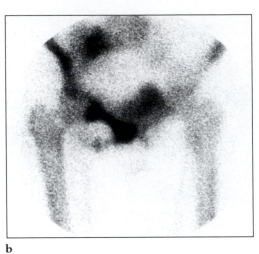

b

# ■ Teaching point

■
A bone scan may detect pelvic fractures which are not seen on X-ray studies.

# Lisfranc's fracture

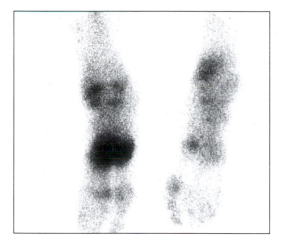

a

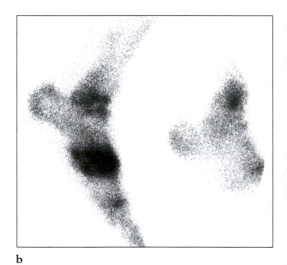

b

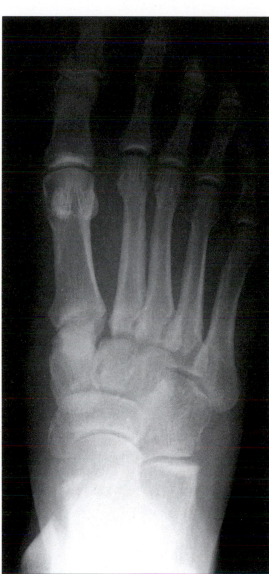

c

**Figure 5.33**

A 35-year-old man who complained of continued right foot pain 2 weeks after a fall, at which time X-ray studies were considered to be normal. Anterior (a) and right lateral (b) bone scans show intense increased tracer uptake extending across the tarsometatarsal articulations (collectively termed Lisfranc's joint) of the right foot. Follow-up X-ray (c) shows a Lisfranc's fracture dislocation of the right mid-foot.

**Figure 5.34**

A 35-year-old man who complained of persistent left foot pain 1 month after a fall. X-rays were normal. The plantar blood pool (a) and both plantar and left lateral (b, c) bone scans show increased vascularity and tracer uptake along the course of Lisfranc's joint. As is frequently the case with a Lisfranc's dislocation, the first tarsometatarsal joint is not involved. Tumour, infection and non-traumatic arthritis do not follow the course of Lisfranc's joint. In this case, a Lisfranc's joint subluxation with spontaneous reduction is the most likely possibility.

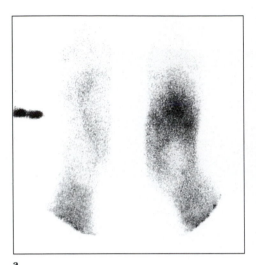

a

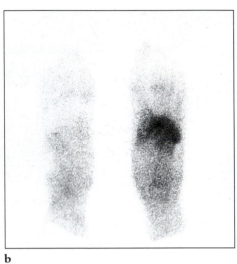

b

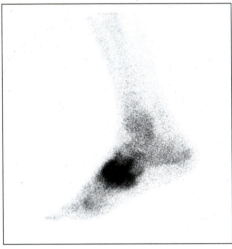

c

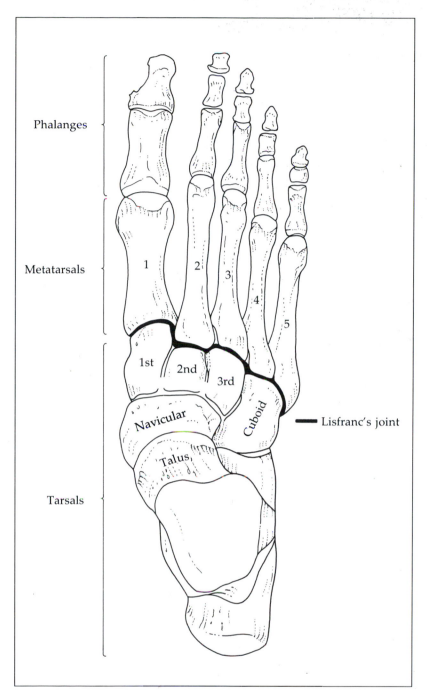

Phalanges

Metatarsals

Tarsals

1

2

3

4

5

1st

2nd

3rd

Navicular

Cuboid

Talus

— Lisfranc's joint

**Figure 5.35**

The 1st to 5th tarsometatarsal joints are collectively referred to as Lisfranc's joint, which is often involved in mid-foot fracture dislocations.

# Growth plate fracture

**Figure 5.36**

A 5-year-old girl who was hit by a lawn mower and sustained a fracture through the distal right femur. While X-ray (a) shows anatomical reduction, there was concern for the viability of the growth plate within the fracture fragment. The bone scan (b) shows no tracer uptake in the fracture fragment, indicating that the involved corner of the growth plate is *not* viable.

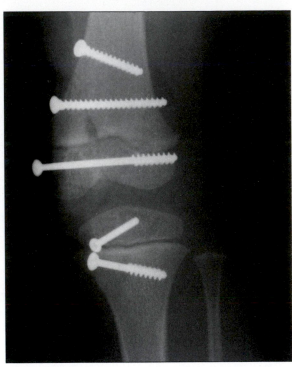

a

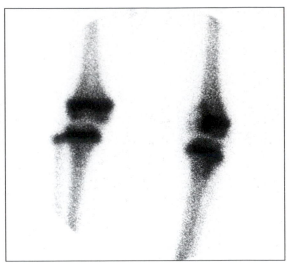

b

# Fracture of femur

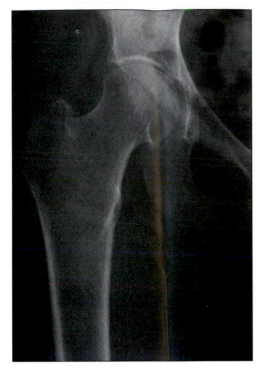

a

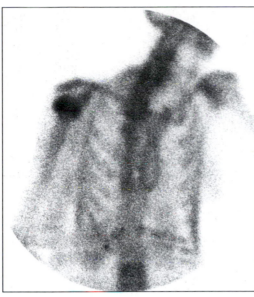

b

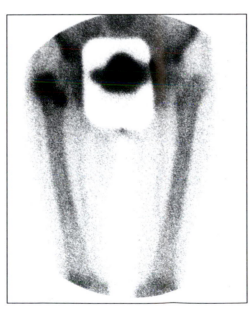

c

**Figure 5.37**

A 79-year-old woman who had suffered a fracture of the anatomical neck of the right humerus 5 days previously, and who refused to walk because of right hip pain. X-ray of the right hip (**a**) shows only an avulsion fracture of the greater trochanter. Bone scans of the right shoulder (**b**) and right hip (**c**) show the humeral fracture and, in addition, indicates an intertrochanteric fracture of the right femur. Internal fixation of the intertrochanteric fracture led to early ambulation and an uneventful recovery.

**Figure 5.38**

Fracture at the neck of the femur. A 56-year-old man who complained of pain in his left hip. **(a)** Bone scan view, anterior pelvis; **(b)** X-ray. The bone scan shows an intense linear area of increased tracer uptake involving the left femoral neck. Scan findings are typically those of fracture of the neck of the femur, which is also shown on X-ray.

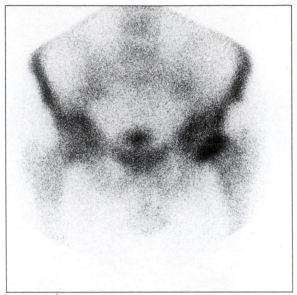

a

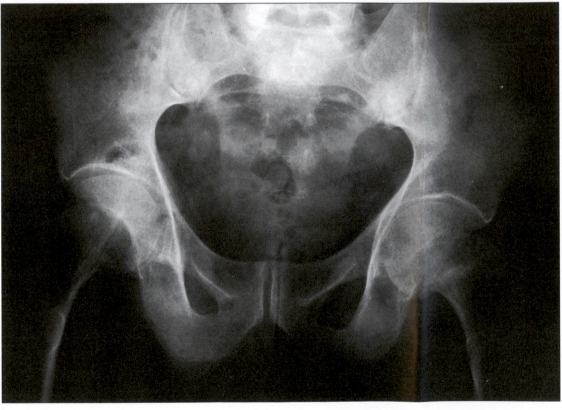

b

# Fracture malalignment

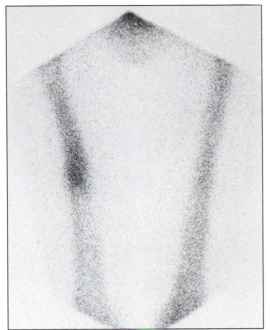

a

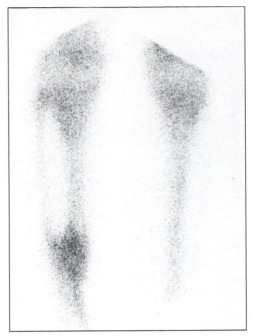

b

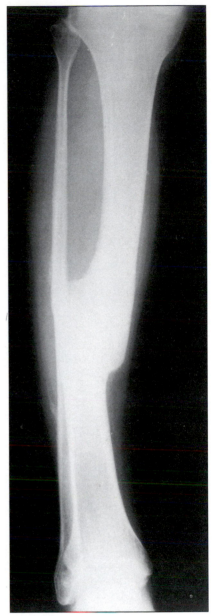

d

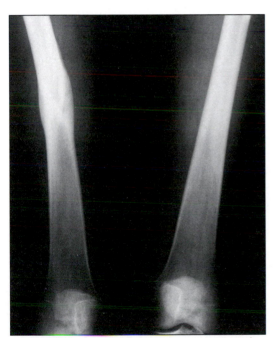

c

**Figure 5.39**

Persistence of activity due to fracture malalignment in a 25-year-old man who sustained a motorcycle injury 10 years previously. Bone scan views of **(a)** femora and **(b)** tibiae and **(c, d)** X-rays. On bone scan images focal abnormalities are present in the mid-right femur and tibia. While the fractures occurred 10 years previously, it is apparent that there is persistent metabolic activity at fracture sites.

## ■ Teaching point

■
When there is malalignment, focal bone scan abnormalities may persist indefinitely.

# Anterior shoulder dislocation

**Figure 5.40**

A 68-year-old man with a history of anterior dislocations of the left shoulder, who complained of recent worsening of his shoulder pain. An anterior view bone scan **(a)** with the humerus in external rotation shows increased tracer uptake about the left shoulder. A 45 degree LPO view **(b)** with the humerus in internal rotation brings the focus of increased activity over the posterolateral aspect of the humeral head into profile. This is the usual site for the Hill–Sachs lesion, a wedge-shaped compression fracture defect caused by recurrent anterior dislocations of the humeral head. In addition, there is increased tracer uptake along the inferior margin of the glenoid which may be due to fracture (Bankart fracture). The X-ray **(c)** confirms the presence of a Hill–Sachs lesion in the left humeral head.

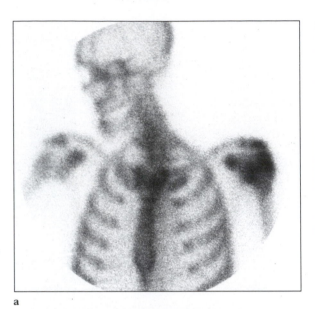

a

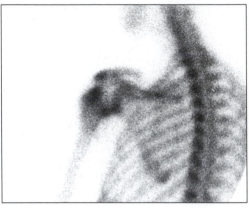

b

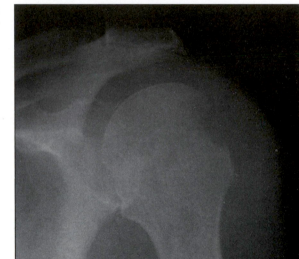

c

# ■ Teaching point

■

The 45 degree posterior oblique view with the humerus held in internal rotation displays the shoulder joint in profile, with no overlap of the humerus and glenoid. This special view aids in recognizing the characteristic findings of recurrent anterior shoulder dislocations.

# Spondylolysis

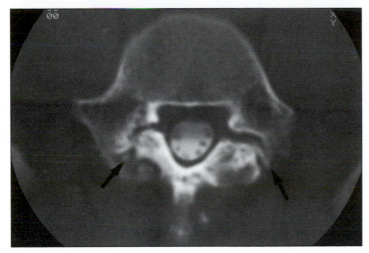

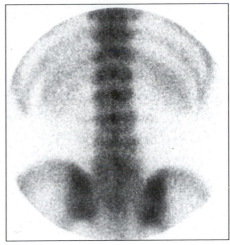

a

b

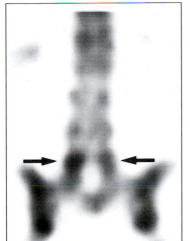

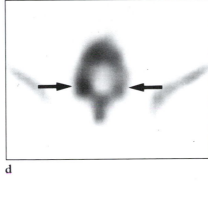

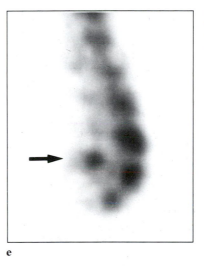

c

d

e

**Figure 5.41**

A 33-year-old man with low back and right leg pain. The CT scan **(a)** shows bilateral L5 spondylolysis (arrows) along with an L4–L5 herniated disc on other CT images that were taken. The planar bone scan **(b)** is normal. The coronal **(c)**, L5 transaxial **(d)**, and sagittal right-of-mid-line **(e)** SPECT bone scans show increased tracer uptake in the region of the pars interarticularis (arrows), which is more pronounced on the right than on the left. The patient was treated with discectomy and L4-to-S1 fusion, with good postoperative pain relief.

**Figure 5.42**

Right-sided L5
spondylolysis in a 52-
year-old man with right-
sided low back pain.
Increased tracer uptake
can be seen on both the
planar **(a)** and transaxial
SPECT **(b)** bone scans in
the region of the right-
sided pars interarticularis
of L5. The bone scan
appearance is not specific
for spondylolysis.
However, the X-ray **(c)**
shows a pars
interarticularis defect at
this site. This
combination of bone scan
and X-ray findings
indicates a metabolically
active spondylolysis
which, in all likelihood, is
the cause of the patient's
low back pain.

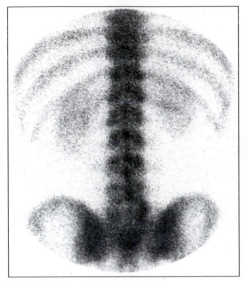

a

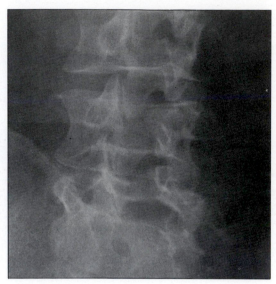

c

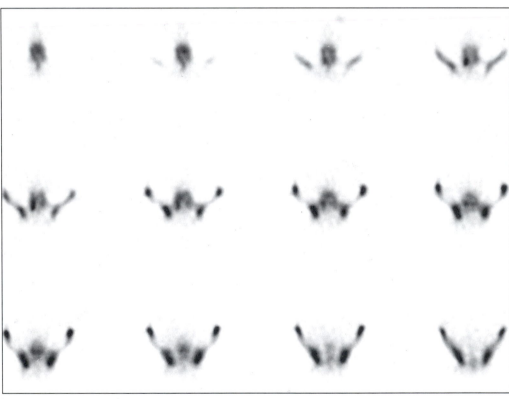

b

# Sports injuries

## Fractures

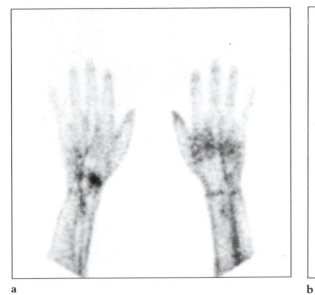

a

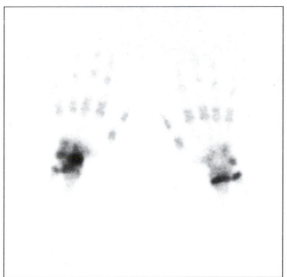

b

**Figure 5.43**

A 16-year-old boy who sustained a right-sided scaphoid fracture while boxing. Bone scan views of hands: **(a)** dynamic, **(b)** delayed image and **(c)** magnified image of right wrist and hand. There is a clear focus of increased tracer uptake in the region of the right scaphoid. This area is highly vascular.

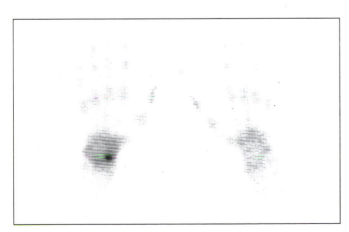

c

**Figure 5.44**

Non-union of fracture. A patient who sustained a fracture of the scaphoid and was still experiencing persistent pain 4 months later. The bone scan shows an intense focus of increased uptake in the region of the scaphoid, attributable to failed union of the fracture.

**Figure 5.45**

A 31-year-old man who sustained multiple cricket ball injuries to the legs while playing cricket 2 weeks previously. Bone scan views: **(a)** dynamic, **(b)** blood pool, **(c)** anterior and **(d)** lateral. Intense foci of increased tracer uptake are seen, associated with the upper left fibula and the medial condyle of the right femur. There is marked increased vascularity to these sites. The scan findings represent fractures.

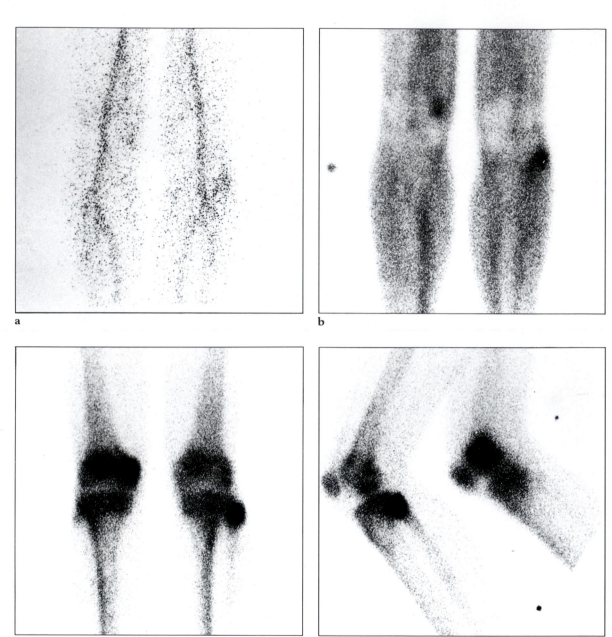

a

b

c

d

# Anterior cruciate ligament tear

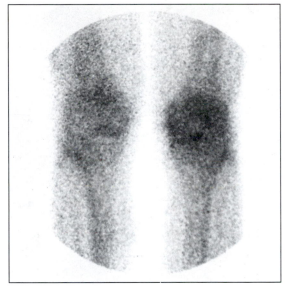

a

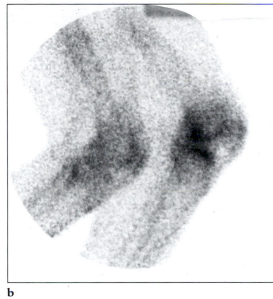

b

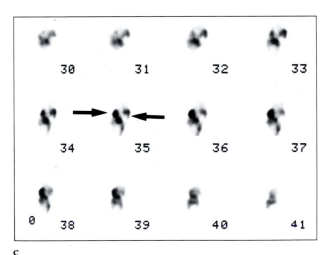

c

**Figure 5.46**

A 65-year-old man who complained of left knee pain 6 months after a hyperextension injury, which had produced a tear of the anterior cruciate ligament. Anterior (**a**) and lateral (**b**) planar bone scan images show increased activity in the left knee. By reviewing sequential sagittal SPECT bone images of the left knee, this activity is easily localized (**c**, arrows) to the origin (medial aspect of the lateral femoral condyle) and insertion (tibial plateau) of the anterior cruciate ligament. X-rays were normal.

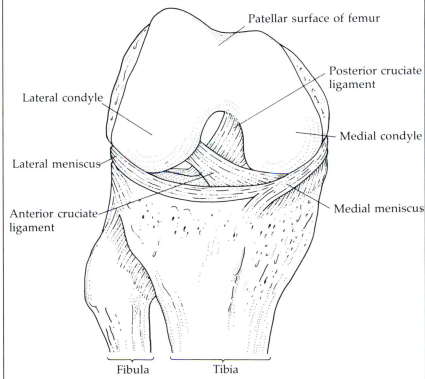

**Figure 5.47**

Anterior and posterior cruciate ligaments are shown on this anterior view of a flexed right knee.

## ■ Teaching point

■

Internal derangements of the knee, including torn menisci and cruciate ligaments, are frequently associated with a focal increase in tracer uptake. While bony damage at the time of the soft tissue injury is one mechanism for this increased tracer uptake, altered joint biomechanics also may be relevant. Following the soft tissue injury, instability or altered joint mechanics will result in increased impact loading on the subchondral bone. This produces a focal osteoblastic response which may appear on bone scan as a site of increased tracer uptake.

# Stress fracture

With the increasing popularity of jogging and other forms of exercise, it is common for patients to complain of pain in a lower limb. While radiography remains the primary diagnostic procedure for identification of skeletal trauma, often the initial X-rays may fail to diagnose an injury. The bone scan may provide valuable information in such cases.

## Table 5.1 Response of bone to increasing stress

| | | *Bone* | *Bone scan/X-ray* | *Symptoms* | *Remodelling* |
|---|---|---|---|---|---|
| S | + | Normal | Normal/Normal | – | Normal: resorption = formation |
| T | | | | | (R)          (F) |
| R | ++ | | ?+ve/Normal | Pain | Accelerated, R>F |
| E | +++ | | +ve/Normal | Pain | Fatigue, R≫F |
| S | | | | | Cortex weakened |
| S | ++++ | | +ve/+ve | Pain | Exhaustion, R≫F |
| | FRACTURE | | | | |

Adapted from Roub LW, Gumerman LW, Hanley EN et al, Bone stress: a radionuclide imaging prospective I, *Radiology* (1979) **132**: 431–438.

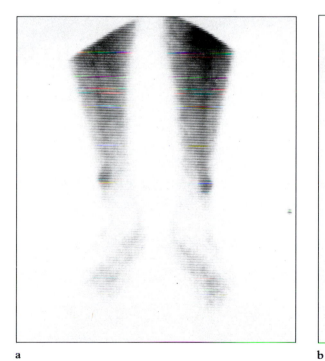

a

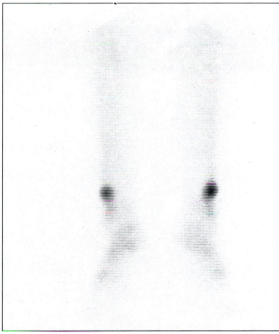

b

**Figure 5.48**

A 20-year-old female ballet dancer with bilateral stress fractures of the fibulae. Bone scan views of lower legs: **(a)** blood pool and **(b)** delayed image. There are focal areas of increased tracer uptake in both lower fibulae just above the ankle. The lesions are highly vascular.

**Figure 5.49**

A 16-year-old female cross-country runner who complained of discomfort in both legs laterally. Bone scan views: **(a)** anterior tibiae in neutral position; **(b)** obtained with internal rotation. There are two focal lesions seen in upper fibulae. However, there is a further lesion which, on anterior view **(a)**, could be in the left mid-tibia, but the internally rotated view **(b)** clearly shows that this is also in the fibula. This patient had multiple fibular stress fractures.

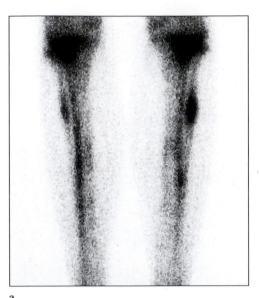

a

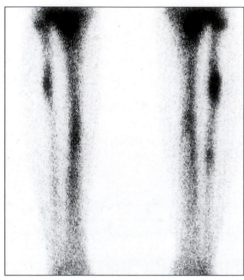

b

# ■ Teaching point

■

Internal rotation views in addition to views with the leg in a neutral position may help to localize lesions in either the tibia or fibula.

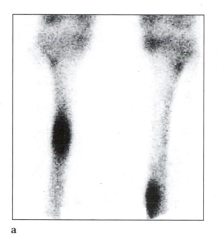

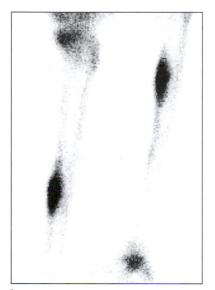

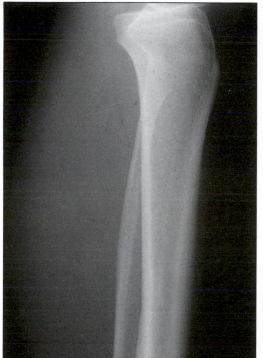

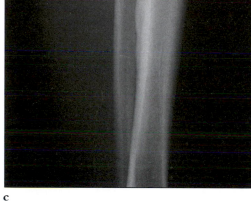

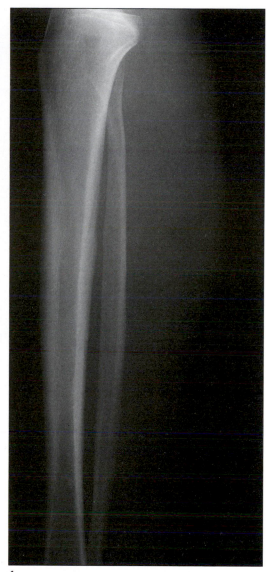

**Figure 5.50**

An 18-year-old female cross-country runner who complained of pain in her calves. Bone scan views: **(a)** anterior tibiae; **(b)** lateral tibiae; **(c, d)** left and right lateral X-rays of tibiae. There are two foci of intensely increased tracer uptake at right mid- and lower third left posterior tibiae. Scan findings are typically those of stress fracture. The intensity of uptake and thickness of lesion differentiate these from shin splints (see Figure 5.65). Initial X-rays were normal, but repeat X-rays 6 weeks later **(c,d)** show intense periosteal reactions, confirming the diagnosis.

## ■ Teaching point

■ Patients with stress fracture may have normal X-rays when they first become symptomatic.

**Figure 5.51**

A 37-year-old jogger who developed pain over the lower left tibia. Bone scan views: **(a)** anterior tibiae and **(b)** lateral. There is a focus of increased tracer uptake in the anterior lower right tibia, extending to the end of the bone. Initial X-rays were normal, but the patient was subsequently shown to have a stress fracture on follow-up X-rays.

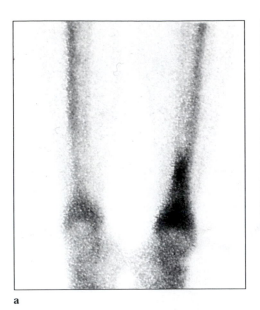
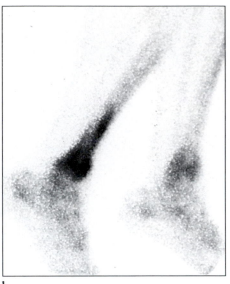

a            b

## ■ Teaching point

■
Stress fractures of proximal or distal long bones on bone scan images often extend to the end of the bone.

**Figure 5.52**

A 30-year-old male jogger. Bone scan views of feet: **(a)** anterior and **(b)** plantar. There is an intense focus of increased tracer uptake seen in the left third metatarsal. This patient had a stress (march) fracture.

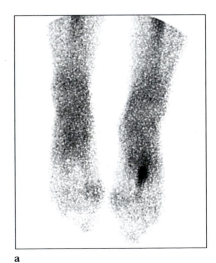
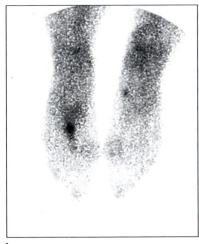

a            b

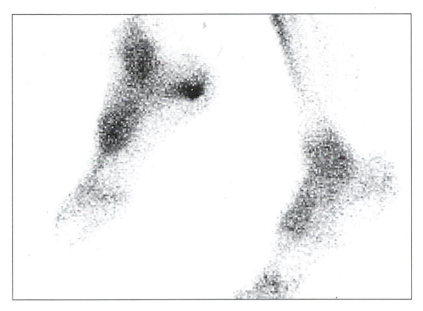

**Figure 5.53**

A 43-year-old woman who complained of pain in her left heel following a tennis match. Bone scan view, lateral feet, shows a focus of increased tracer uptake along the plantar surface of the left calcaneus. The diagnosis was plantar fasciitis.

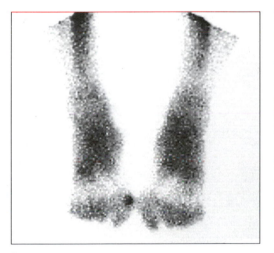

a

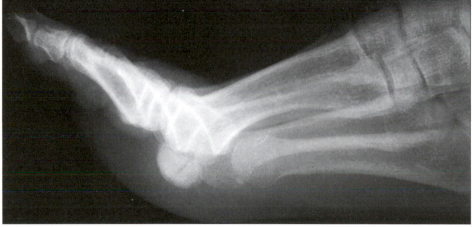

b

**Figure 5.54**

A 30-year-old woman jogger who complained of pain in her right foot. **(a)** Anterior bone scan view of the feet and **(b)** right lateral foot X-ray. An intense focus of tracer uptake is seen in the region of right first metatarsal head. This corresponds to a fracture in a sesamoid bone seen on X-ray.

## ■ Teaching point

■

While sesamoid bones may be bipartate, the positive bone scan indicates significant alteration in skeletal metabolism and confirms healing of the fracture.

**Figure 5.55**

Bilateral L4 pars interarticularis stress fractures. This 20-year-old American football player complained of increasingly severe low back pain. X-rays, including oblique views, were normal. The posterior planar bone scan **(a)** shows increased tracer uptake over both the left and right sides of L4. This abnormality is better localized on the transaxial SPECT image through the L4 vertebra **(b)**. The patient gave up vigorous sports, and the low back pain disappeared.

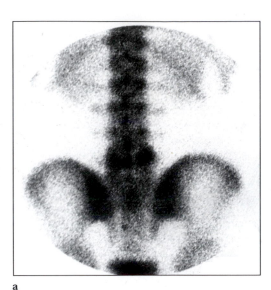

a

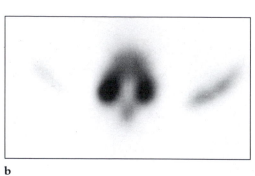

b

**Figure 5.56**

A 32-year-old jogger with right hip pain and normal X-rays. The bone scan view of the anterior pelvis, shows a focus of increased tracer uptake in the right calcar femorale. This patient had a femoral stress fracture.

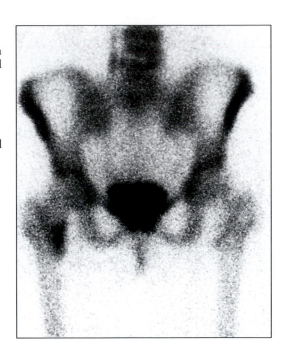

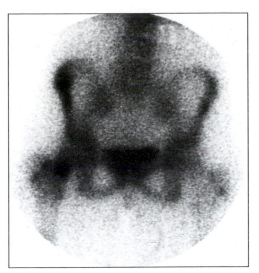

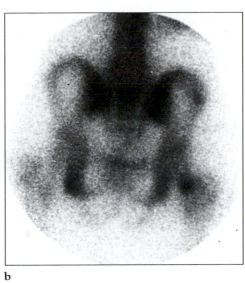

a

b

**Figure 5.57**

An 18-year-old female jogger who complained of pain in her right groin. Bone scan views: **(a)** anterior and **(b)** posterior pelvis. There is a small, intense focus of increased tracer uptake seen at the medial cortical margin of the right femoral neck. With normal X-rays this indicates the presence of a stress fracture.

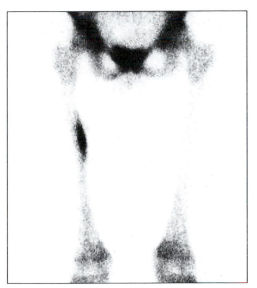

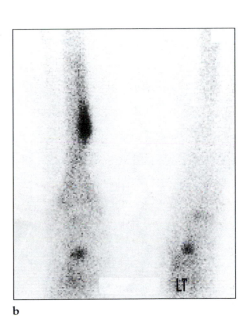

a

b

**Figure 5.58**

A 16-year-old jogger and aerobics dancer. Bone scan views: **(a)** anterior femora and **(b)** anterior lower tibiae, obtained 2 years later. This patient initially complained of pain in the right thigh and was shown to have a stress fracture of the femur; 2 years later, the patient presented with pain in the right lower leg, and was shown to have a tibial stress fracture.

**Figure 5.59**

A 16-year-old ballet dancer with a stress fracture. Bone scan views of lower legs: **(a)** original study and **(b)** 10 months later. There is a focal lesion present at the medial aspect of the right lower tibia, caused by a stress fracture. On the repeat study, the lesion has resolved.

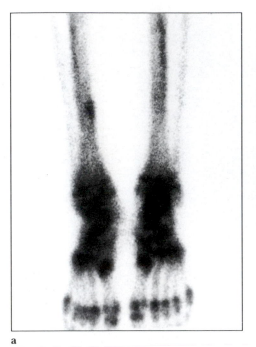
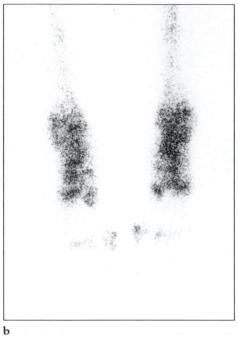

a

b

**Figure 5.60**

A 24-year-old male weightlifter with a stress fracture of the humerus. Bone scan views: **(a)** right arm and **(b)** left arm. There is increased tracer uptake throughout both humeri, particularly at the lower medial aspects. The linear changes at this site are typical of periosteal reaction, and the scan appearances in the humeri presumably reflect cortical hypertrophy. In addition, there is a focus of more intense increased tracer uptake at the medial aspect of the upper third of the left humerus, indicating a stress fracture.

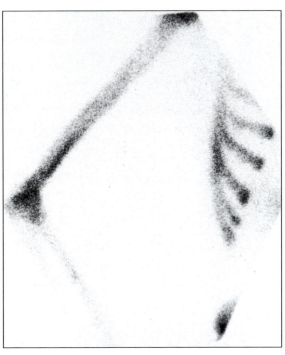
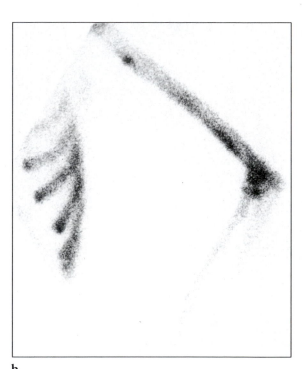

a

b

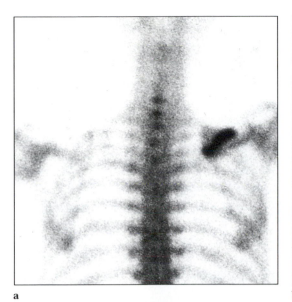

a

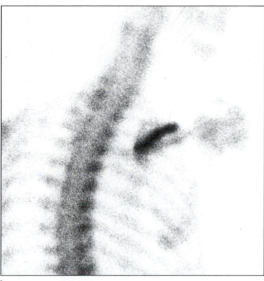

b

**Figure 5.61**

A 25-year-old male jogger, who was running with weights in both hands. Bone scan views: **(a)** upper posterior thoracic spine, and **(b)** right posterior oblique. **(c)** X-ray of the right shoulder. There is a linear intense area of increased tracer uptake extending obliquely across the right scapula. The X-ray confirms the presence of a fracture (arrow).

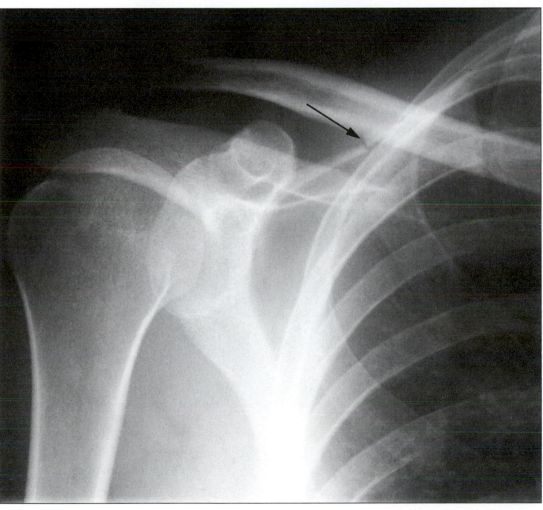

c

**Figure 5.62**

A 37–year-old left-handed man who plays basketball and racquetball and who, in addition, uses a sledgehammer at work, complained of left shoulder discomfort. Bone scan views: **(a)** anterior right shoulder and **(b)** left shoulder. **(c)** X-ray of left shoulder. There is an intense focus of increased tracer uptake seen in the region of the left acromioclavicular joint. Note the slight subluxation of the distal end of the left clavicle when compared with the normal right side.

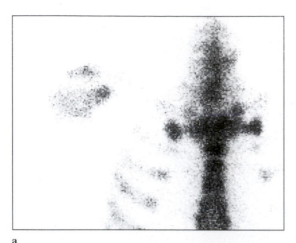

a

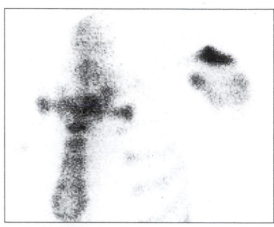

b

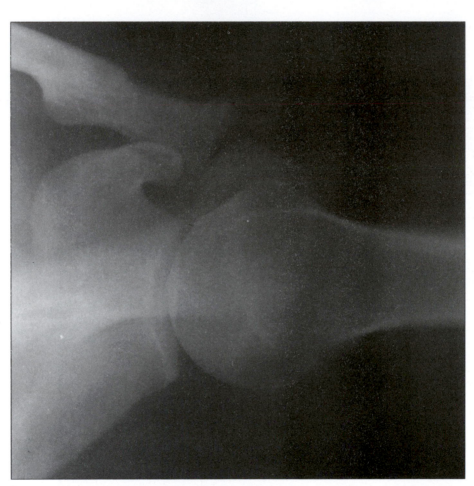

c

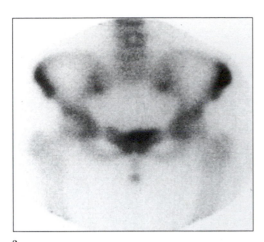

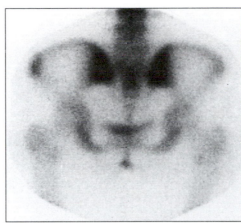

a                    b

**Figure 5.63**
A 60-year-old female runner, who had complained for several months of left anterior hip pain. Bone scan views: **(a)** anterior pelvis and **(b)** posterior pelvis. **(c)** X-ray of pelvis. There is increased tracer uptake in the region of the left anterior iliac crest. The X-ray shows separation of the apophysis, which is typical of a traction injury.

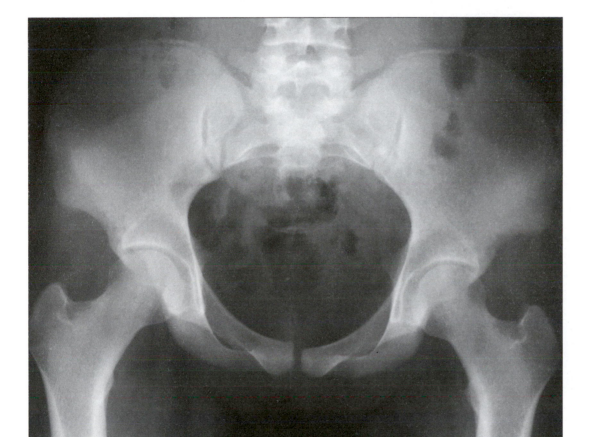

c

**Figure 5.64**

A 47-year-old man with a past history of a twisting injury to his leg 3 years previously, who complained of difficulty in walking. Bone scan views: **(a)** dynamic anterior hips and **(b)** delayed anterior pelvis. **(c)** X-ray of left hip. There is an intense focus of increased tracer uptake adjacent to the right femoral neck. There is increased vascularity to the soft tissue at this site. The X-ray, which was initially interpreted as normal, shows subtle density changes of myositis. This diagnosis was confirmed surgically.

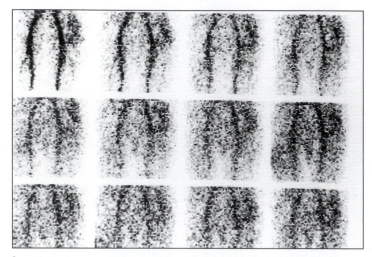

a

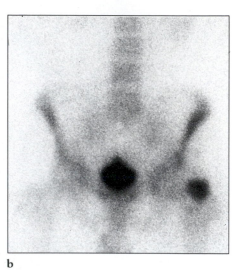

b

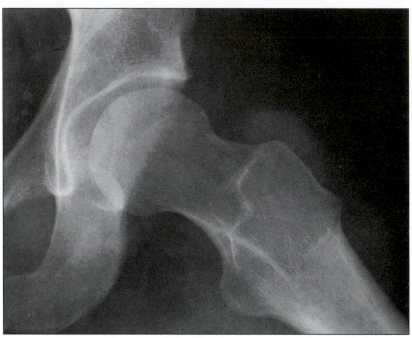

c

# Shin splints

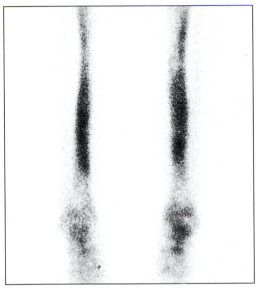

a

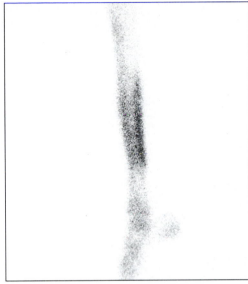

b

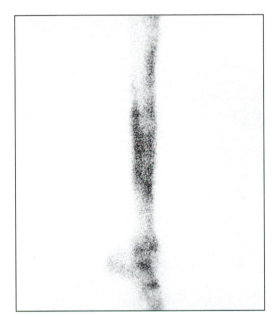

c

**Figure 5.65**

A 26-year-old aerobics teacher with shin splints. Bone scan views of tibiae: **(a)** anterior, **(b)** right lateral and **(c)** left lateral. There is strikingly increased tracer uptake diffusely along the posterior third of both tibiae and, in addition, there is some increased tracer uptake throughout the rest of the tibiae. Note also slightly increased tracer uptake in the left forefoot. The scan appearances of the posterior tibiae are typical of shin splints. The more generalized increased tracer uptake in the tibiae presumably reflects cortical hypertrophy. The scan appearances in the left forefoot are non-specific but are likely to represent minor degenerative changes.

## ■ Teaching points

■
Differentiation between shin splints and stress fracture is important. Shin splints is a syndrome which is due to a periosteal reaction at the site of muscle insertion at the lower third of the posterior tibia. Patients can continue with exercise as long as they feel comfortable. However, patients with stress fracture must avoid exercise for at least 6 weeks, as they are at risk of sustaining complete fracture.

■
It is important to obtain lateral views in patients who are complaining of pain in a lower limb, as otherwise the diagnosis of shin splints will be missed.

# Benign bone tumours

## Osteoid osteoma

**Figure 5.66**

Bone scan views of femora: **(a)** blood pool and **(b)** delayed image. **(c)** X-ray of the upper left femur. There is a discrete focus of increased tracer uptake seen in the upper third of the left femur. The lesion is vascular. This corresponds to the lucency seen on the X-ray, representing a central nidus. The overall appearances are typical of an osteoid osteoma.

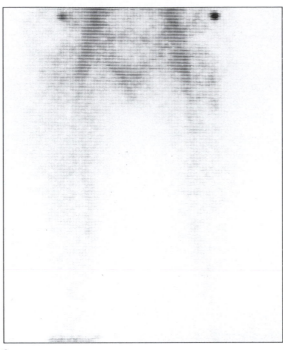

a

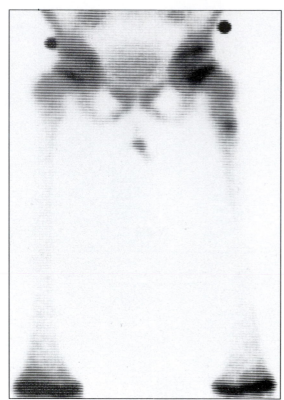

b

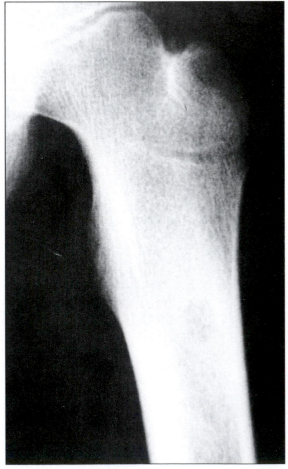

c

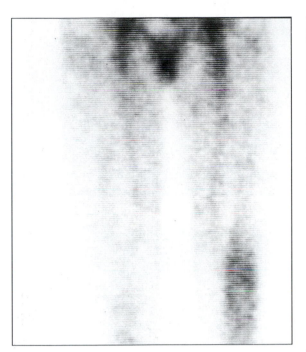

a

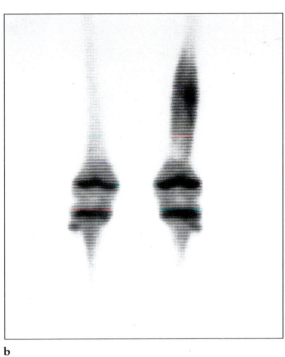

b

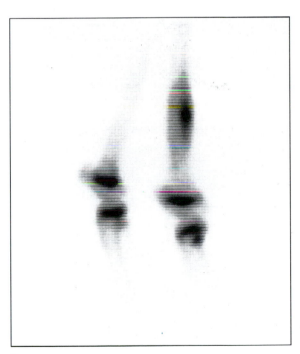

c

**Figure 5.67**

A further case of osteoid osteoma involving a femur. Bone scan views of lower femora and knees: **(a)** blood pool, **(b)** anterior and **(c)** lateral. There is increased blood flow and increased tracer uptake in the left lower femur, which corresponded to an area of intense periosteal reaction seen on an X-ray. On the bone scan, it is apparent that a more focal area of increased tracer uptake is seen within the generalized lesion. When an osteoid osteoma arises in the mid-shaft of a long bone, there may be an intense cortical reaction which can occasionally be confused with a malignant bone tumour.

**Figure 5.68**

Further cases of osteoid osteoma. **(a, b)** Osteoid osteoma of the left calcaneus. **(c, d)** Osteoid osteoma of the hamate bone.

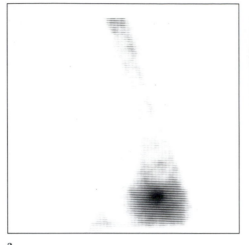

a

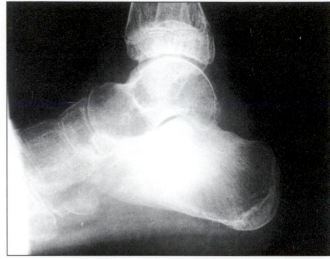

b

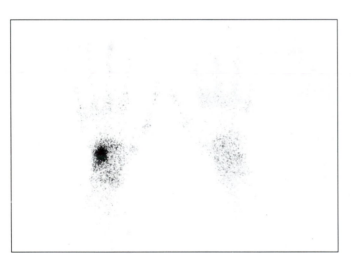

c

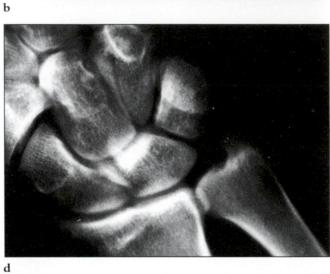

d

**Figure 5.69**

A contrast-enhanced CT scan **(a, b)** shows a calcified lesion adjacent to the inner table of the left frontal bone. Likely diagnostic possibilities include osteoma and meningioma. Bone scan **(c)** shows active uptake of tracer by the lesion which favours the diagnosis of osteoma rather than a small meningioma. The dynamic phase of a $^{99m}$Tc–DTPA brain scan **(d)** along with 2 hour delayed images **(e)** show no increased vascularity or breakdown in the blood–brain barrier. Once again, the scan findings favour osteoma rather than meningioma.

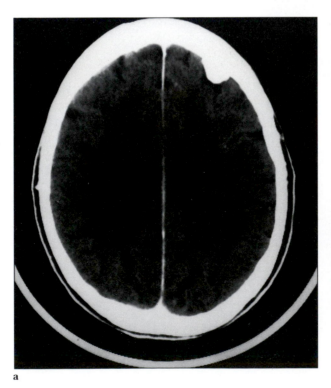

a

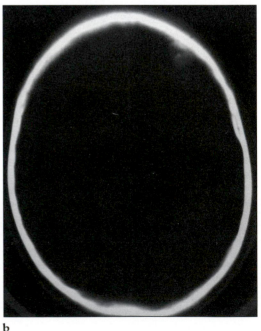

b

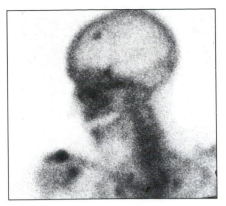

c

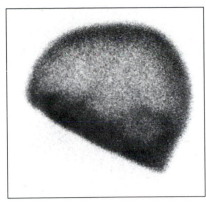

e

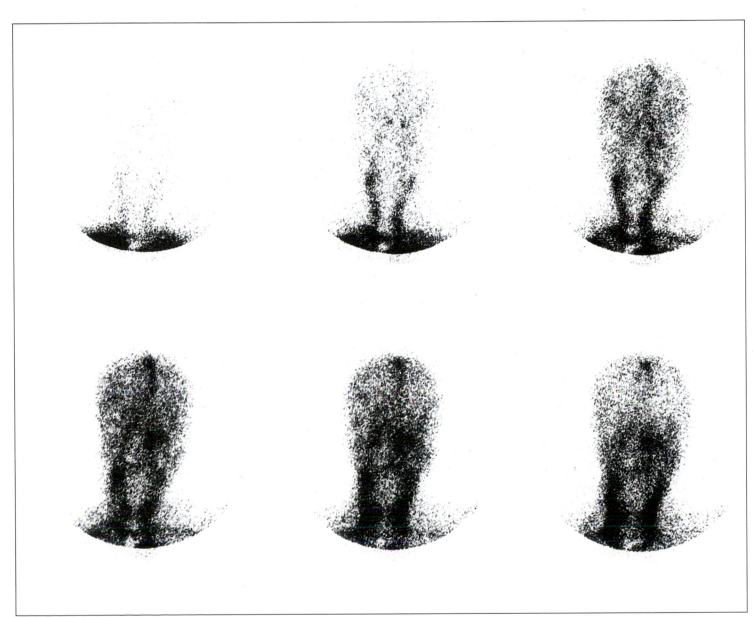

d

**Figure 5.70**

A 36-year-old man with low back pain. Conventional X-ray studies were normal. The posterior view planar bone scan **(a)** shows increased activity over the left side of L5, that is well localized to the bony posterior neural arch on the transaxial **(b)** and coronal **(c)** SPECT images. The CT scan **(d)** shows an osteoid osteoma adjacent to the left-sided superior articular facet of S1.

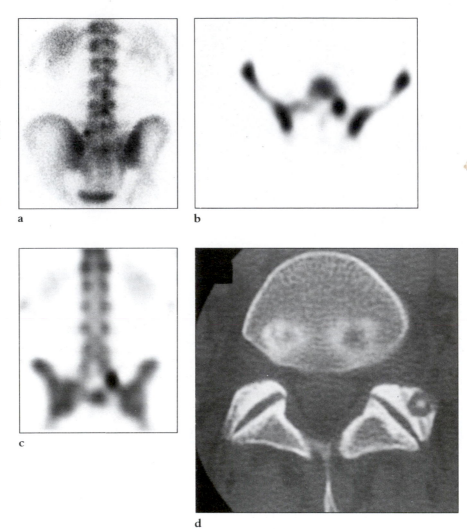

a

b

c

d

# Aneurysmal bone cyst

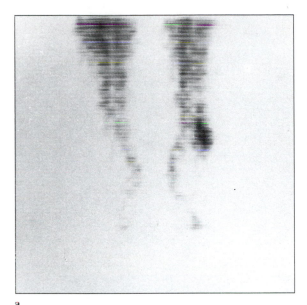

a

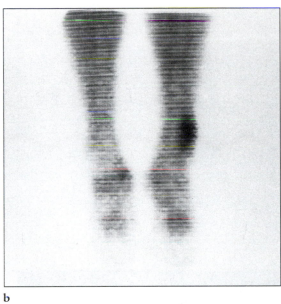

b

**Figure 5.71**
Bone scan views of lower limbs: **(a)** dynamic, **(b)** blood pool and **(c)** delayed; **(d)** X-ray of the left lower tibia/fibula. There is a focus of increased tracer uptake associated with the lower left fibula, which has a relatively photopaenic central area. There is increased vascularity and blood pool to this site. Scan findings were due to an aneurysmal bone cyst, which is seen on X-ray. However, it is apparent that the lesion is metabolically active.

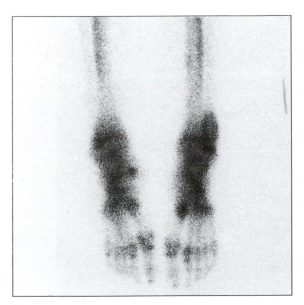

c

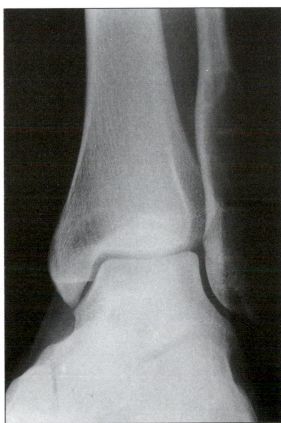

d

# Enchondromatosis

**Figure 5.72**

A 40-year-old man known to have enchondromatosis. Multiple bone scan images including views of the hands **(a)** and tibiae **(b)** show evidence of increased tracer uptake and anatomical deformity, with closely matching radiographic findings **(c, d)**.

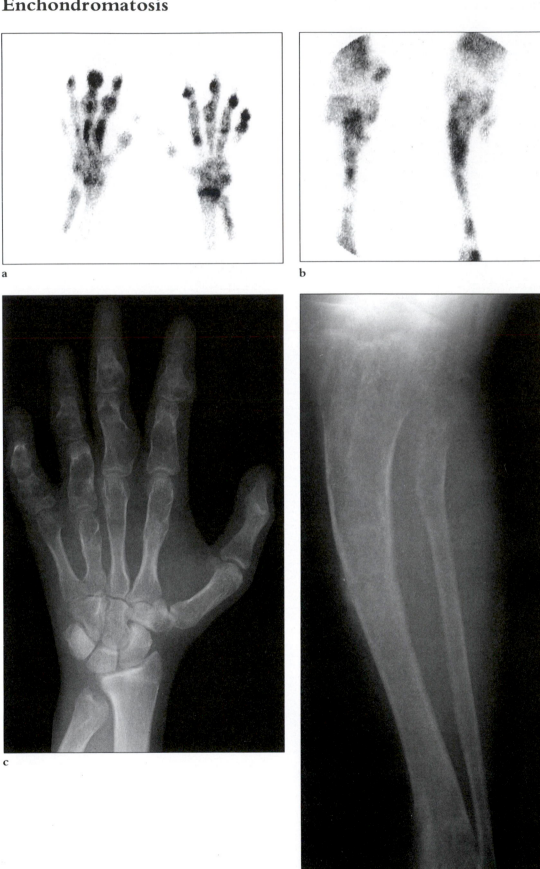

# Meningioma

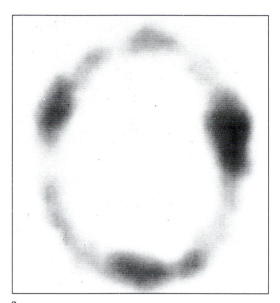

a

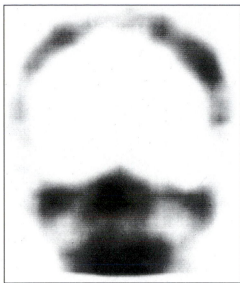

b

**Figure 5.73**

A 53-year-old woman who complained of headache. There is a focal area of increased tracer uptake in the left frontal bone, which is seen on transaxial (a) and coronal (b) SPECT but not planar (c) bone scan images. A contrast-enhanced CT scan demonstrated a probable meningioma adjacent to the inner table of the skull at this site. The meningioma incited a minimal increase in metabolism within the calvarium, which was detected on the SPECT bone scan.

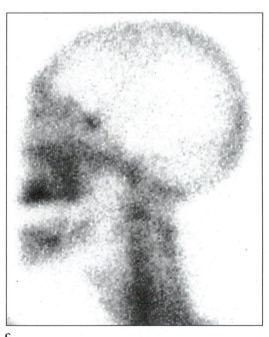

c

# Ivory osteoma

**Figure 5.74**

A 32-year-old male acromegalic with an ivory osteoma. Bone scan views of skull: **(a,d)** left lateral and **(b,e)** anterior. An intense focus of increased tracer uptake is seen in the left supraorbital area **(a, b)**. This appearance is typical of an ivory osteoma, which was confirmed on X-ray **(c)**. This patient subsequently complained of severe pain in the left frontal region of the skull. The repeat bone scan **(d, e)** shows, in addition to the above, increased tracer uptake extending upwards and laterally, involving the frontal sinus. The scan findings were due to sinusitis.

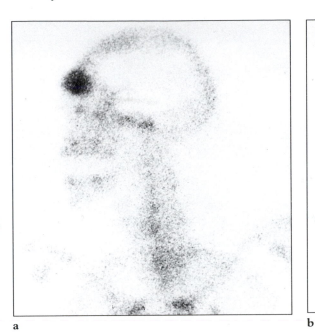

a

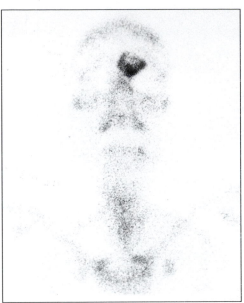

b

c

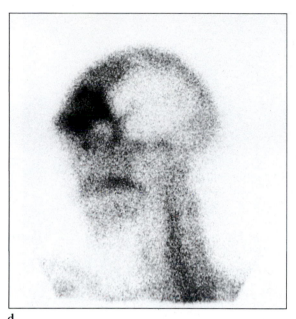

d

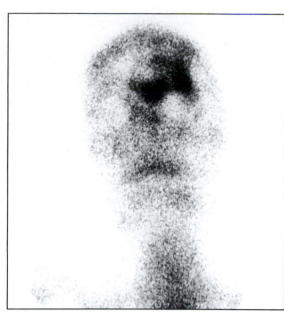

e

# Haemangioma of the spine

**Figure 5.75**

A 34-year-old man with haemangioma of the spine. **(a)** Bone scan view of posterior thoracic spine and **(b)** corresponding X-ray. There is a slight reduction of tracer uptake diffusely throughout the body of T11 (arrow). This corresponds to the changes seen on the X-ray, which are those of haemangioma.

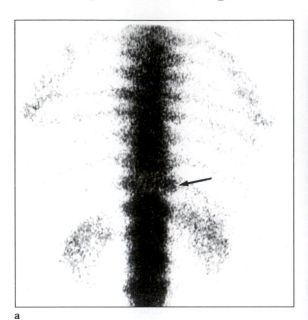

a

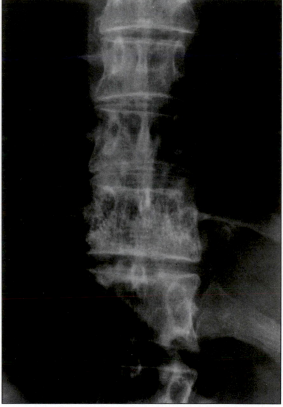

b

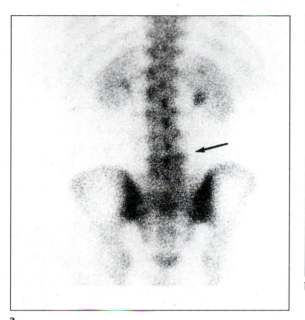

a

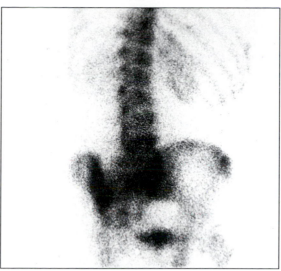

b

**Figure 5.76**

A 37-year-old man with haemangioma. Bone scan views: (a) posterior lumbar spine and (b) right posterior oblique. (c) X-ray. There is slightly increased tracer uptake throughout L4 (arrow) corresponding to the changes of haemangioma seen on the X-ray.

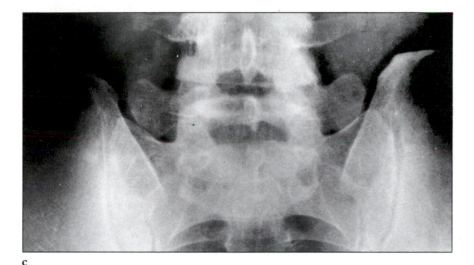

c

## ■ Teaching point

■
Haemangioma of the spine may appear either photon-deficient or show slightly increased tracer uptake on the bone scan study.

# Infection

The standard diphosphonate bone scan and imaging with gallium-67 ($^{67}$Ga) and indium-111 ($^{111}$In)-labelled white cells have been used to identify osteomyelitis and to differentiate it from cellulitis. A triple-phase bone scan should always be obtained in cases of suspected infection. Acute osteomyelitis is characterized by increased vascularity and enhanced activity in the delayed skeletal images, whereas cellulitis shows increased vascularity but normal or low-grade bone uptake on delayed images.

In some cases, the diagnosis may still be in doubt, and a $^{67}$Ga or $^{111}$In-labelled white cell scan will provide additional information. There is some controversy as to which is the more sensitive investigation. The indium study will identify the sites of active white cell migration and, while more specific for infection, has a higher false negative rate, particularly in patients being treated with antibiotics. Gallium-67 has bone-seeking properties in its own right, and will show uptake at any areas of increased metabolic activity. This study should be read in conjunction with the bone scan image, and features which strongly favour infection are:

- Focally increased uptake greater than that seen on the corresponding bone scan image, or
- Focally increased uptake which does not correspond precisely to a discrete lesion on the bone scan.

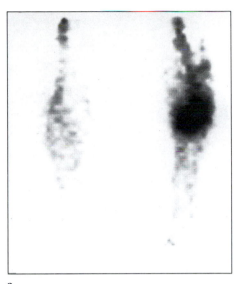

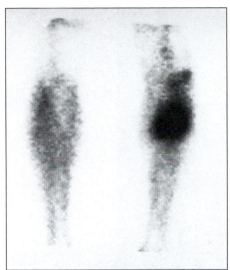

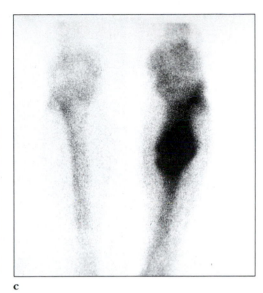

a

b

c

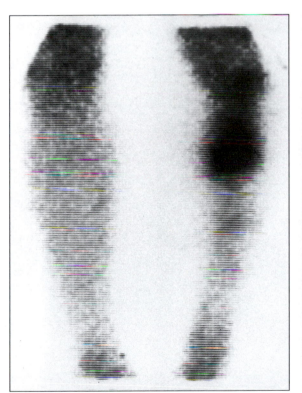

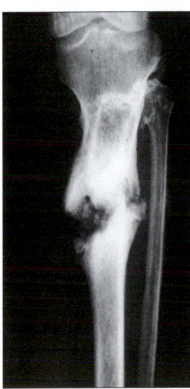

d

e

## Figure 5.77

A 44–year–old man with a fractured tibia, non–union and infection. Bone scan views of tibiae: **(a)** dynamic, **(b)** blood pool, **(c)** delayed image and **(d)** gallium scan. **(e)** X-ray. On the bone scan views there is marked vascularity to the upper third of the left tibia, and on the delayed image there is strikingly increased tracer uptake at that site corresponding to both ends of the fracture. On the gallium scan there is strikingly increased tracer uptake in the region of the non–united fracture.

# Non-union without infection

**Figure 5.78**

A reactive non-union in an old fracture of the distal tibial diaphysis (**a**, X-ray) produces an oblique band of increased tracer uptake on bone scan (**b**). This is probably the site where the unhealed fracture margins meet with bony impact loading that stimulates an osteoblastic response. Infection was considered as a possible cause for non-union. However, the $^{67}$Ga scan (**c**) shows only minimal tracer uptake at this site, suggesting that osteomyelitis was not present.

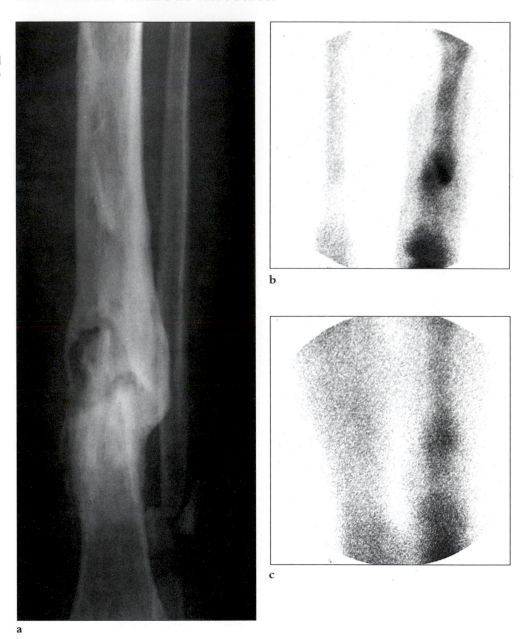

a

b

c

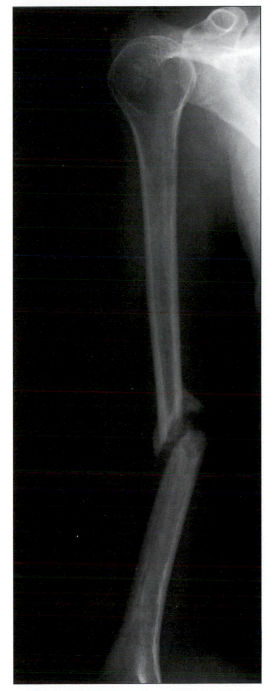

a

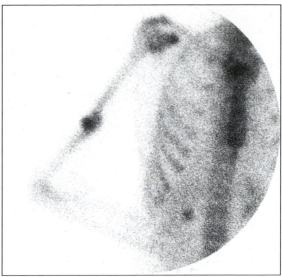

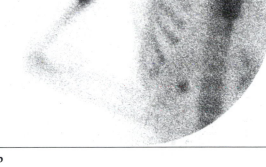

b

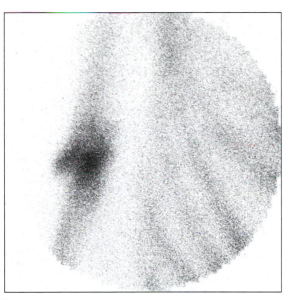

c

**Figure 5.79**

A 35-year-old man who had continued pain 1 year after fracture of the right humerus. The X-ray **(a)** shows no evidence of bridging callus at the fracture site. Both a routine bone scan image **(b)** of the right humerus and an oblique magnified bone scan image **(c)** were obtained. While the fracture site appears 'hot' on **(b)**, on the magnified image a break within the increased uptake at the fracture site is clearly seen. Even with electrical stimulation of bone it is unlikely that the fracture will heal. Subsequent bone grafting produced a solid union.

## ■ Teaching point

■

This case demonstrates the use of bone scanning to distinguish between delayed union and non-union. The break within the increased uptake at the fracture site indicates deficient callus formation. Even when using high resolution bone scanning techniques, multiple images including anterior, posterior, lateral and oblique views may be required.

# Osteomyelitis

**Figure 5.80**

An elderly diabetic patient who had previous amputation of the right great toe. Bone scan views of both feet: **(a)** blood pool and **(b)** delayed image. The right foot was painful and swollen. The bone scan shows intense metabolic activity with increased vascularity at the site of amputation. Subsequent investigations confirmed osteomyelitis.

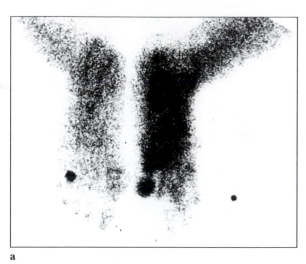

a

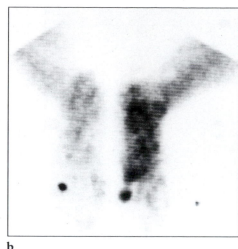

b

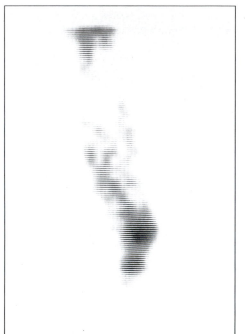

a

b

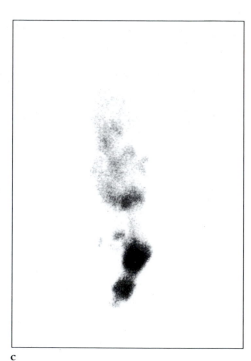

c

**Figure 5.81**

A further case of osteomyelitis of the foot in a diabetic patient. Bone scan views: **(a)** dynamic, **(b)** blood pool and **(c)** delayed. The bone scan shows vascular inflammatory lesions involving the left great toe.

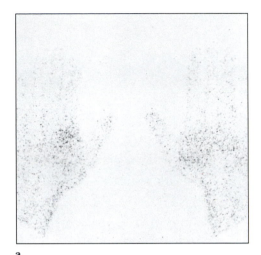

a

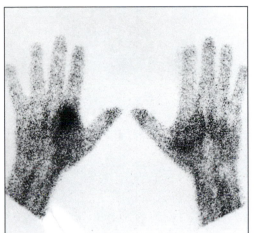

b

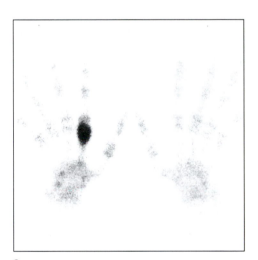

c

**Figure 5.82**

Bone scan views of hands:
(a) dynamic, (b) blood
pool and (c) delayed. (d)
X-ray. There is an intense
focus of increased tracer
uptake seen in the
proximal second
metacarpal. There is
increased vascularity at
this site, and the X-ray
shows a periosteal
reaction. The scan
findings were due to
osteomyelitis.

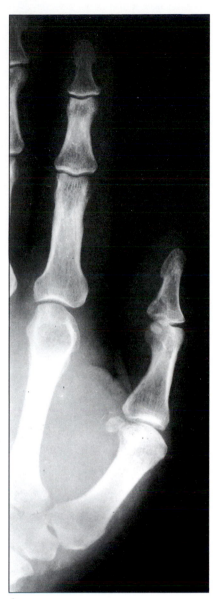

d

**Figure 5.83**

A 13-year-old boy with right ankle pain. The anterior blood pool image **(a)** shows increased vascularity in the distal right tibia. The anterior bone scan image **(b)** shows increased tracer uptake at the same site. The X-rays were normal. Culture results confirmed the diagnosis of osteomyelitis.

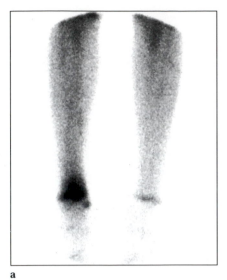

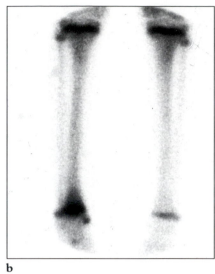

a

b

**Figure 5.84**

A 6½-year-old girl who complained of pain in her right thigh. Bone scan views of femora: **(a)** dynamic and **(b)** delayed image. There is increased tracer uptake in the right upper femur. This area is vascular. This child had confirmed osteomyelitis of the right femur.

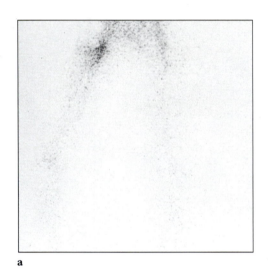

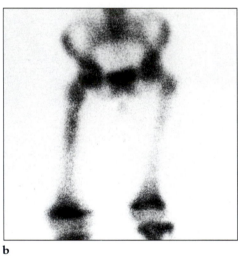

a

b

**Figure 5.85**

A 49-year-old man who presented with an enlarging submental mass associated with a draining sinus. Anterior and lateral bone scans **(a, b)** show increased tracer uptake in the left side of the mandible.
*(Continued)*

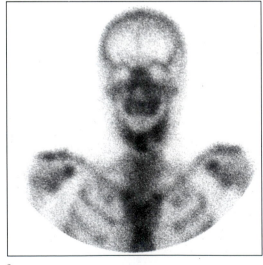

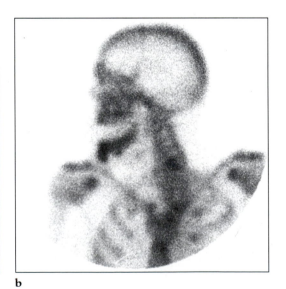

a

b

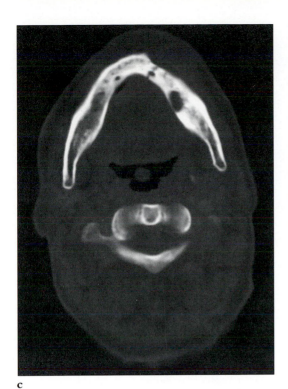

c

**Figure 5.85** *continued*

There is a photon-deficient area within this zone of increased uptake which corresponds to an area of bone destruction on the CT scan (c) from which actinomycosis was cultured. Anterior (d) and lateral (e) $^{67}$Ga images show avid tracer uptake in the bone abscess. Note also the $^{67}$Ga uptake in the submental draining sinus.

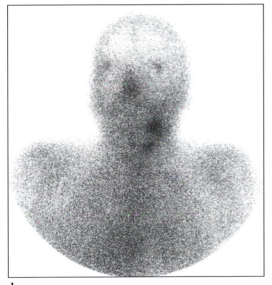

d

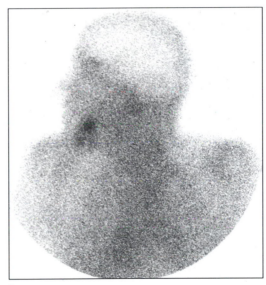

e

**Figure 5.86**

A 23-year-old man who had continued pain and swelling 8 months after a segmental fracture of the mandible. The X-ray **(a)** shows non-union at the junction of the fracture fragment and the right side of the mandible. In such cases, if osteomyelitis can be excluded, bone grafting is the treatment of choice for this non-union. Anterior **(b)** and right lateral **(c)** bone scans show tracer uptake about the fracture margins, which is non-specific and could be explained by continuing bony repair rather than osteomyelitis. A photopaenic defect is present at the site of non-union. Anterior **(d)** and right lateral **(e)** ⁶⁷Ga images show no significant uptake in the mandible, which argues strongly against osteomyelitis. Cultures obtained at the time of bone grafting were negative.

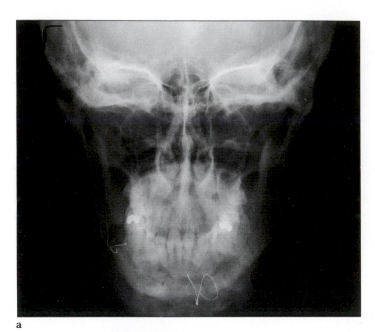

a

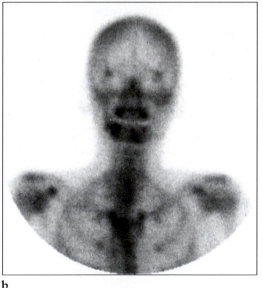

b

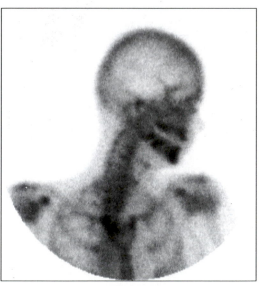

c

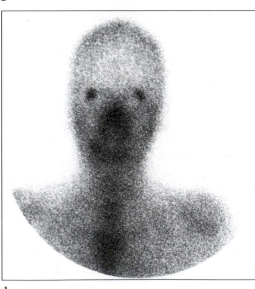

d

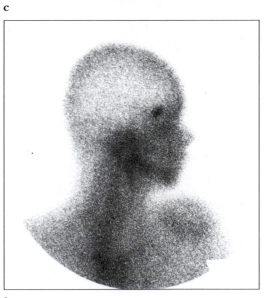

e

# Multifocal osteomyelitis

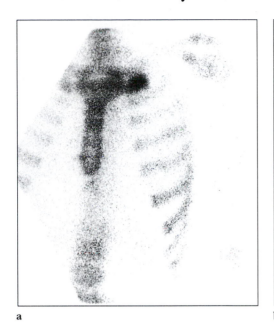

a

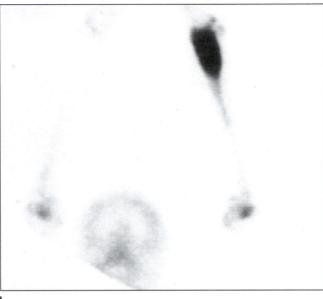

b

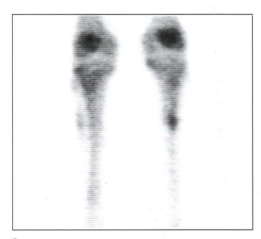

c

**Figure 5.87**

A 34-year-old man with osteomyelitis. Bone scan views: **(a)** left anterior chest, **(b)** forearms and **(c)** anterior tibiae. **(d)** X-ray of left forearm. There is an extensive focus of increased tracer accumulation at the distal end of the left radius. In addition, there are foci of increased activity at the medial end of the first left rib, upper left tibia and right fibula. The X-ray of the forearm shows a lytic lesion of the distal left radius, with extensive periosteal reaction. Note that the presence of multifocal disease made a diagnosis of osteomyelitis perhaps more likely than a primary bone tumour involving the radius.

## ■ Teaching points

■
Osteomyelitis may be multifocal.

■
A whole body scan should be obtained routinely.

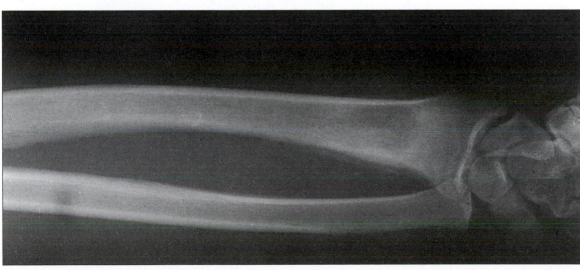

d

**Figure 5.88**

Bone scan views of femora: **(a)** blood pool, **(b)** delayed image and **(c)** following antibiotic therapy. **(d)** X-ray of left femur. There is strikingly increased tracer uptake to the lower third of the left femur, and also in the medial aspect of the left tibial plateau. These areas are highly vascular. Following antibiotic therapy, the scan appearances show marked improvement, with resolution of the tibial abnormality. The initial bone scan appearances in isolation are suggestive of Paget's disease, but are in fact due to an acute exacerbation of chronic osteomyelitis. Once again, this case makes the point that the bone scan is sensitive but the appearances are non-specific.

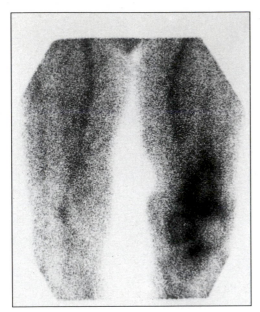

a

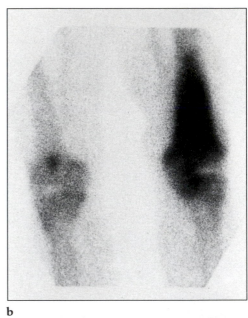

b

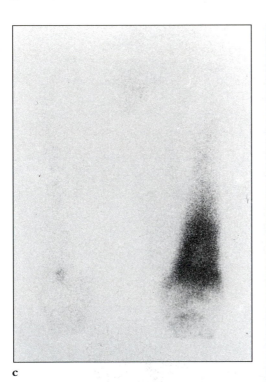

c

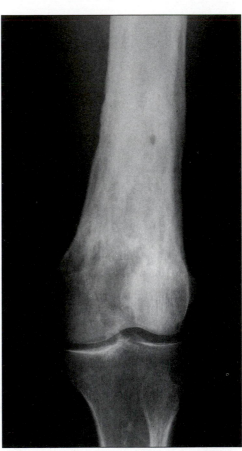

d

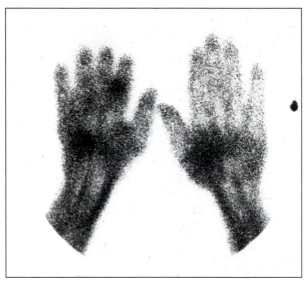

a

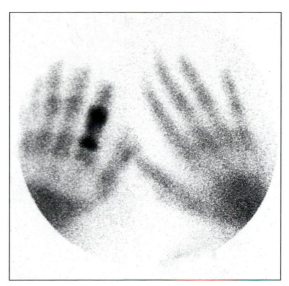

b

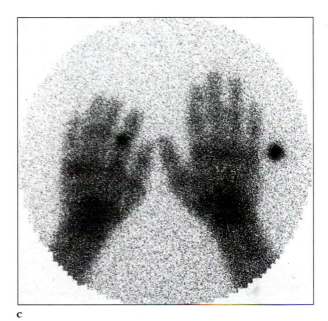

c

**Figure 5.89**

A 34–year-old man who suffered a penetrating injury to the left second PIP joint. X-ray studies 3 weeks later showed soft tissue swelling without fracture. The blood pool scan **(a)** shows a generalized increase in vascularity throughout the left hand, which is most pronounced at the left 2nd PIP. The bone scan **(b)** shows increased tracer uptake throughout the proximal phalanx, which is most intense at the ends of the bone. The $^{67}$Ga scan **(c)** shows focal intense uptake confined to the region of the left second PIP joint. This discordance between the distribution of intense uptake on bone and $^{67}$Ga scans is strongly suggestive of infection. Joint aspiration confirmed the diagnosis of septic arthritis.

## ■ Teaching point

■

Differences in the relative distributions of $^{99m}$Tc–MDP and $^{67}$Ga uptake suggest significant infection. This is particularly true if the $^{67}$Ga uptake involves a larger area and/or is more intense than the zone of increased $^{99m}$Tc–MDP uptake.

# Treated osteomyelitis

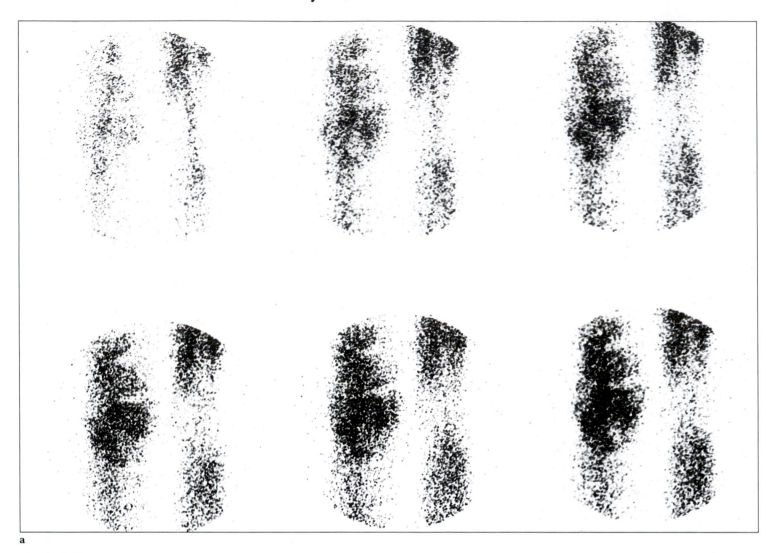

a

**Figure 5.90**

A 21-year-old man with an open fracture of the right knee and distal femur began to drain pus from his wound site. The dynamic flow study **(a)** and anterior bone scan of the knees **(b)** show increased vascularity and bony repair, which can all be accounted for by the recent fracture and insertion of the metallic external fixator. The anterior $^{67}$Ga image **(c)** shows intense uptake, indicating osteomyelitis and significant soft tissue infection. Following 4 months of parenteral antibiotic therapy, a repeat dynamic study **(d)** shows a slight decrease in vascularity in the right thigh, probably representing muscle wasting. The anterior bone scan **(e)** shows less active bony repair in the femoral diaphysis with continued intense tracer uptake near the right knee. The follow-up $^{67}$Ga scan **(f)** shows no abnormal uptake along the shaft of the right femur and adjacent soft tissues consistent with cure of the infection. $^{67}$Ga uptake around the right knee is less intense than the activity seen on bone scan and is probably secondary to bony repair rather than infection. Based in part on the bone and $^{67}$Ga scan findings, antibiotics were discontinued. Infection did not recur.

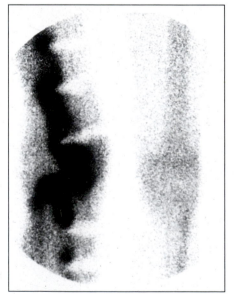

b

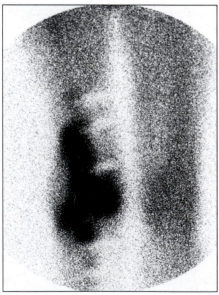

c

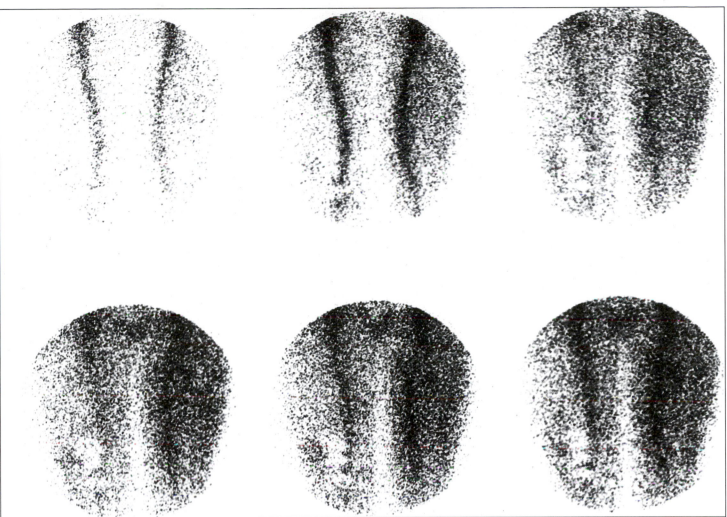

d

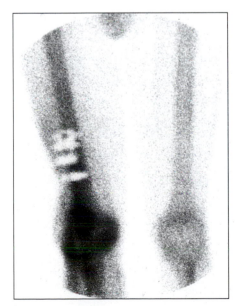

e

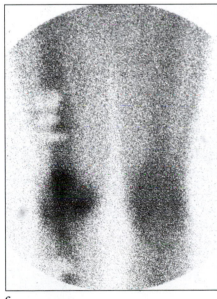

f

## ■ Teaching point

■ When treating osteomyelitis, the results of sequential [67]Ga scans may influence the decision to discontinue antibiotic therapy. However, the interpretation of [67]Ga scans is complicated by the tendency for the tracer to localize at all sites of increased osteoblastic activity. Therefore, a bone scan for comparison with the [67]Ga images is often obtained. When acute osteomyelitis has been successfully treated, the [67]Ga scans will usually either return to normal or will show bony uptake which is much less intense than the uptake of $^{99m}$Tc-MDP.

# Osteomyelitis revealed by $^{67}$Ga SPECT

**Figure 5.91**

A 30-year-old woman who presented with back pain which was eventually shown to be due to tuberculosis. Bone scan view **(a)** shows increased tracer uptake at T10 and T11 which was the site of the patient's pain. Anterior **(b)** and posterior **(c)** planar $^{67}$Ga scans show normal activity in the liver which in part obscures the lower thoracic spine. A sagittal SPECT $^{67}$Ga scan **(d)** directly through the mid-line shows active tracer uptake in the lower thoracic spine (straight arrow), which lies posterior to activity within the left lobe of the liver (curved arrow). The X-ray **(e)** shows disc space narrowing and vertebral body endplate destruction at the T10/T11 level.

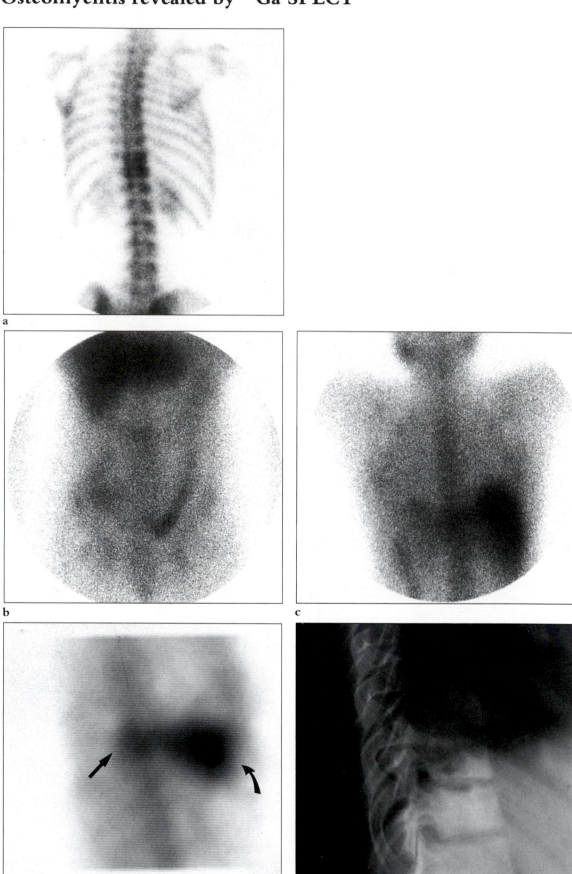

# Arthritis

## Osteoarthritis

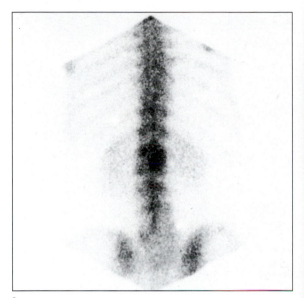

a

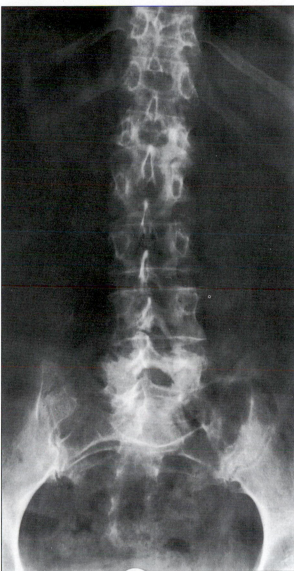

b

**Figure 5.92**

A 70-year-old woman who complained of pain in her back. **(a)** Bone scan view of the lumbar spine; **(b)** corresponding X-ray. There is a focal area of increased tracer uptake at the right border of L1/2. The scan appearances are non-specific but represent degenerative change, which is confirmed on the X-ray.

**Figure 5.93**

**(a)** Bone scan view of the posterior lumbar spine; **(b)** corresponding X-ray. There is a focus of increased tracer uptake seen at the left aspect of L2/3, which extends beyond the normal anatomical border. The X-ray reveals a large osteophyte at that site.

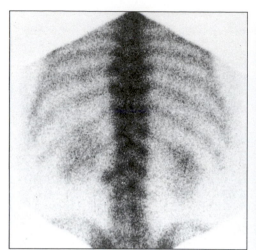

a

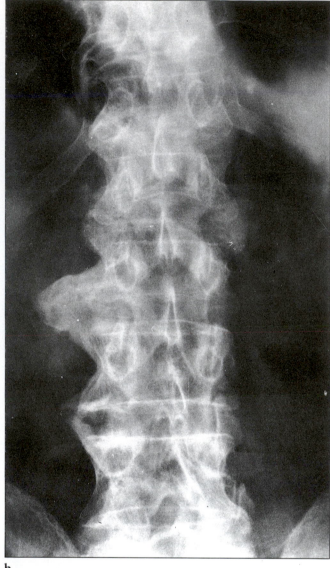

b

## ■ Teaching point

■ Note that not all sites of degenerative change are seen on the bone scan. A positive scan result depends on metabolic activity, and inactive lesions, ie, 'burnt–out' disease, will not be visualized.

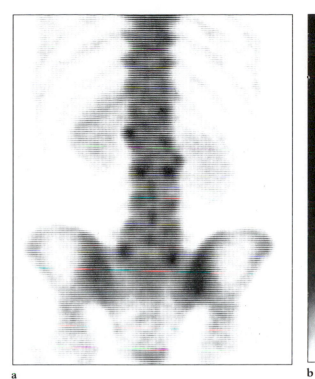

a

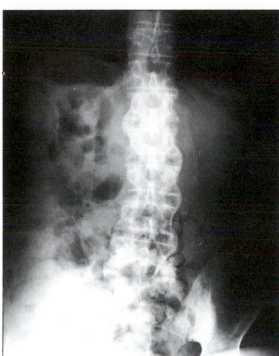

b

**Figure 5.94**

(a) Bone scan, posterior view of the lower thoracic and lumbar spine; (b) corresponding X-ray. In this case, multiple focal areas of increased tracer uptake are present in the lumbar spine at the following sites: left border of L1/2, corresponding to a large osteophyte seen on the X-ray; right L2/3 junction, again corresponding to an osteophyte; L3 pedicles; L5/S1 articulations bilaterally and symmetrically. This patient had carcinoma of the breast and had a bone scan as part of routine evaluation. Although focal abnormalities are present in the spine, they are all attributable to degenerative change, with no evidence of metastatic disease.

**Figure 5.95**

A 40-year-old woman with degenerative change secondary to congenital dislocation of both hips. **(a)** Bone scan view of anterior pelvis and upper femora; **(b)** X-ray. There are metabolically active lesions involving both femoral heads. Scan findings are consistent with X-ray changes, which demonstrate severe degenerative disease which was secondary to congenital dislocation of both hips.

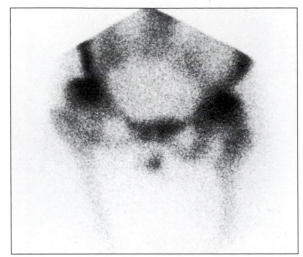

a

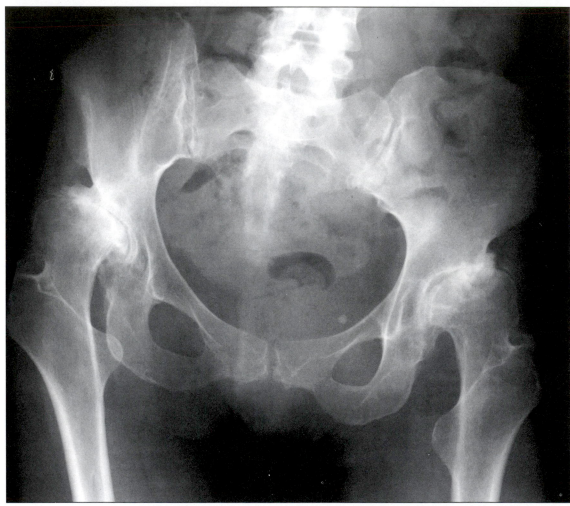

b

# Articular facet osteoarthritis

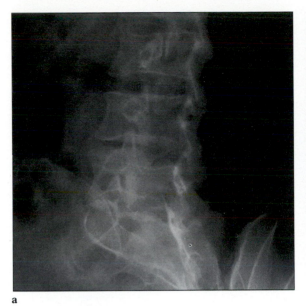

a

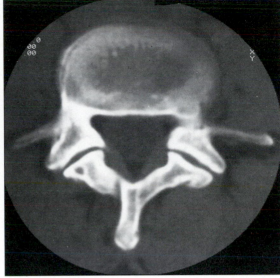

b

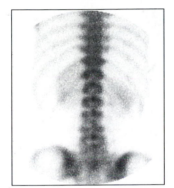

c

**Figure 5.96**

A 30-year-old woman who complained of low back and right leg pain. The X-ray **(a)** and CT scan **(b)** show minimal osteoarthritis of the right-sided L4/L5 articular facet. The planar bone scan **(c)** is normal. Coronal SPECT bone scans **(d)** show increased activity over the right side of the bony posterior neural arch in the region of the right-sided L4/L5 articular facet (arrow). Diagnostic articular facet block confirmed L4/L5 facet disease as the cause of low back pain. Introduction of a needle into this articular facet exacerbated the back pain, and the injection of a local anaesthetic and steroids produced complete pain relief.

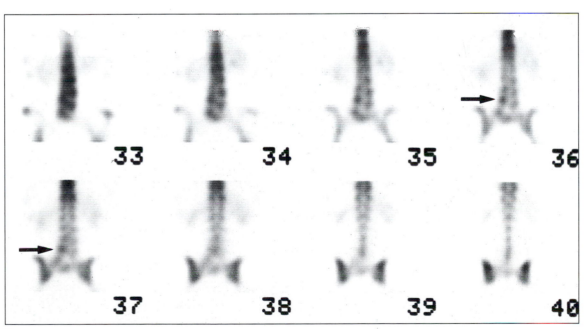

d

**Figure 5.97**

Another case of painful articular facet disease on coronal **(a)** and L5 transaxial **(b)** SPECT bone scans. The bone scan findings in this 59-year-old woman with low back pain are not specific. Other possibilities include spondylolysis or bone metastases. Correlation with clinical findings, X-ray, CT, diagnostic articular facet injection or, rarely, even biopsy may be needed to arrive at a specific diagnosis.

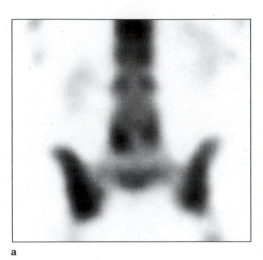

a

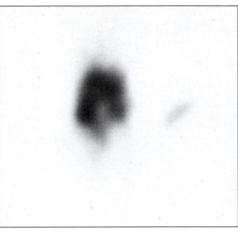

b

# Schmorl's node

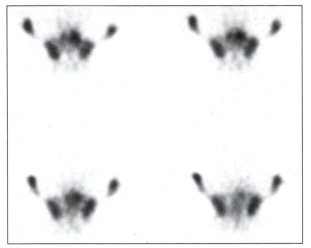

a

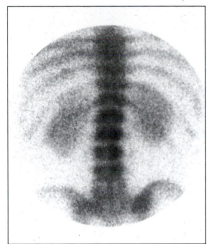

b

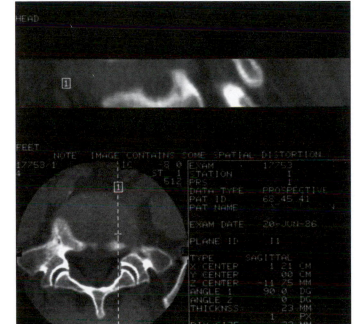

c

**Figure 5.98**

A 55-year-old man with intermittent low back pain showed evidence of increased uptake over the left side of the L5 vertebral body on transaxial SPECT images **(a)** which was not evident on the posterior planar bone scan **(b)**. Conventional X-ray studies were normal. CT scans reformatted into the sagittal plane **(c)** demonstrated a sclerotic bony reaction at the site of a Schmorl's node. This is probably an incidental finding rather than the cause of the patient's intermittent low back pain.

# 'Hot' patella sign

**Figure 5.99**

**(a)** Bone scan, anterior view, of the knees; **(b)** X-ray of left lateral knee. Both patellae show marked uptake of tracer on the bone scan images. The X-ray reveals that increased uptake is due to degenerative change.

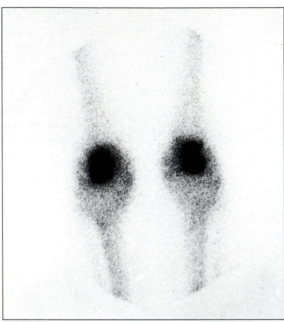

a

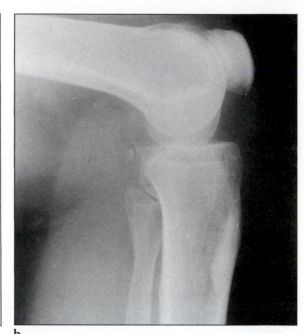

b

# Lateral patellar facet osteoarthritis

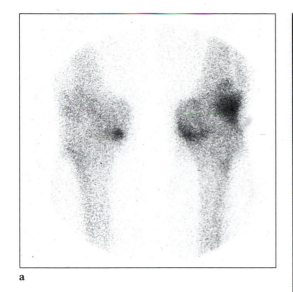

a

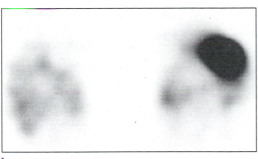

b

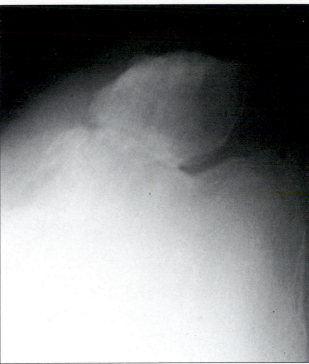

c

**Figure 5.100**

A 70-year-old man who complained of progressive left knee pain. An anterior planar bone scan **(a)** and a transaxial SPECT image through the patellae **(b)** show intense uptake over the lateral aspect of the left patella. Also present on the planar scan are the typical findings of moderately advanced medial compartment osteoarthritis. X-ray **(c)** confirmed osteoarthritis of the lateral patellar facet. Resection and drilling of the lateral patellar facet provided pain relief and improved function.

# Patellar avulsion fracture

**Figure 5.101**

An avulsion fracture of the lower pole of the right patella in a 16-year-old boy who developed knee pain while running. Bone scan views of knees: **(a)** anterior and **(b)** right lateral. A focus of increased tracer uptake is seen at lower aspect right patella which corresponds to the fracture seen on the X-ray **(c)**.

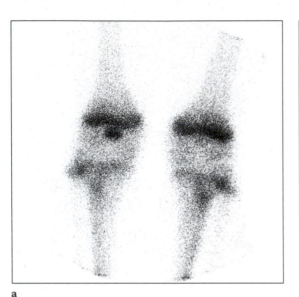

a

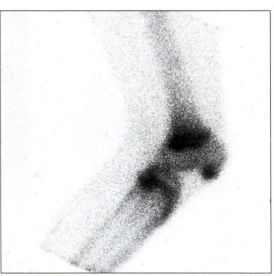

b

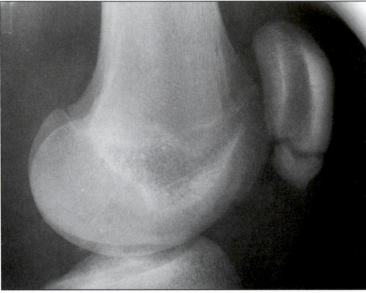

c

# Arthritis of the hands

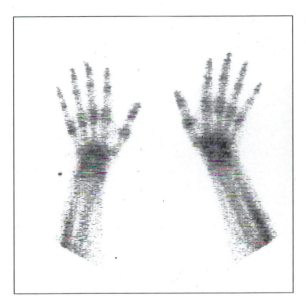

**Figure 5.102**

Normal hands.

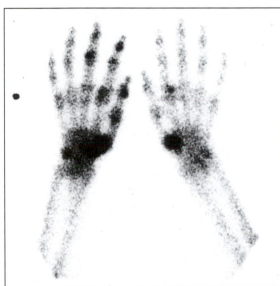

**Figure 5.103**

Osteoarthritis. Multiple focal areas of increased tracer uptake are present in the interphalangeal joints, particularly involving the distal joints. There is bilaterally increased tracer uptake at the first carpometacarpal joint. The scan appearances are typically those of osteoarthritis.

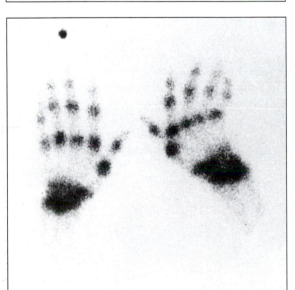

**Figure 5.104**

Rheumatoid arthritis. There is increased uptake of tracer in both wrists, with more focally increased uptake in many small joints of the hands. Ulnar deviation is apparent. The scan appearances are typical of rheumatoid arthritis.

**Figure 5.105**

Osteoarthritis of the hands. Bone scan views: **(a)** blood pool and **(b)** delayed. On the blood pool view there is increased tracer accumulation at the right 3rd, 4th and 5th PIP joints, and the left 1st interphalangeal joint and the 2nd proximal interphalangeal joint. On delayed views there is also increased tracer uptake in all of the interphalangeal joints, and also the metacarpal phalangeal joint of the first digits bilaterally and the ulna-styloid region on the left. While the delayed images are typical of osteoarthritis, it is apparent that there is some inflammatory component to this arthritic process.

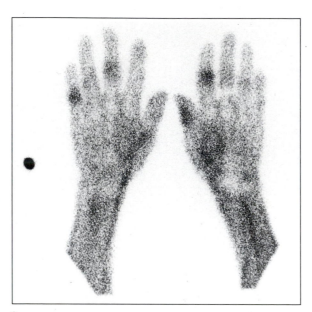

a

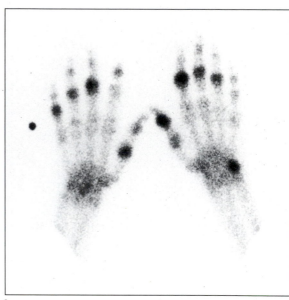

b

## ■ Teaching point

■
Osteoarthritis may have a significant inflammatory component.

# Rheumatoid arthritis

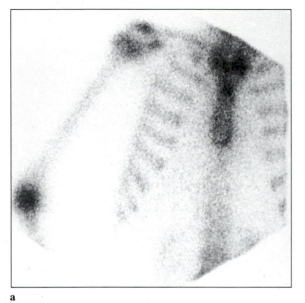

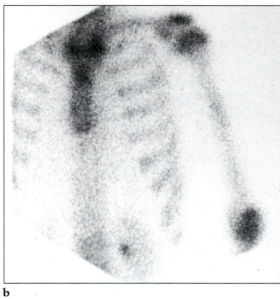

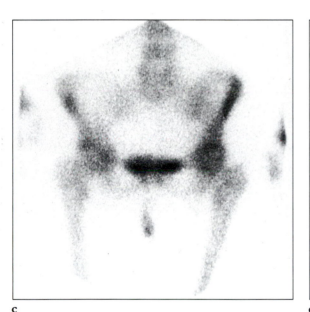

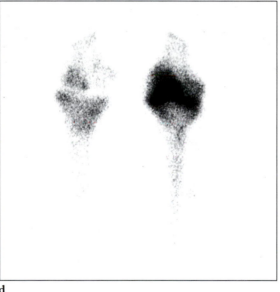

a

b

c

d

**Figure 5.106**

Bone scan views: **(a)** anterior right chest, **(b)** anterior left chest, **(c)** anterior pelvis and **(d)** knees. There is increased tracer uptake in association with both shoulders, elbows, and knees (more marked on the left), and the left hip. Scan findings were attributable to rheumatoid joint disease.

## Sacroiliitis

The bone scan is more sensitive than routine radiography for the detection of early sacroiliitis, as illustrated in Figure 5.107.

**Figure 5.107**

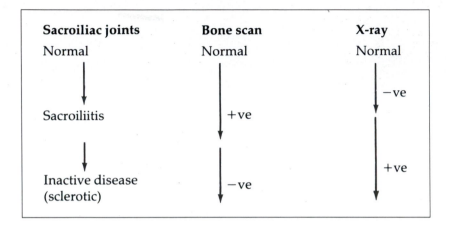

| Sacroiliac joints | Bone scan | X-ray |
|---|---|---|
| Normal | Normal | Normal |
| ↓ | | −ve ↓ |
| Sacroiliitis | +ve ↓ | |
| ↓ | | +ve ↓ |
| Inactive disease (sclerotic) | −ve ↓ | |

Visual assessment of tracer uptake in the sacroiliac joints is difficult, and quantitation is recommended. Several different methods have been proposed, one of which is shown in Figure 5.108.

**Figure 5.108**

Sacroiliac joint quantitation.

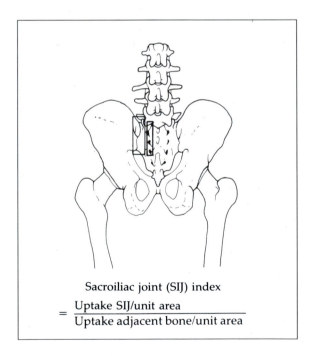

Sacroiliac joint (SIJ) index

$$= \frac{\text{Uptake SIJ/unit area}}{\text{Uptake adjacent bone/unit area}}$$

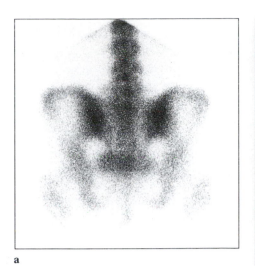

a

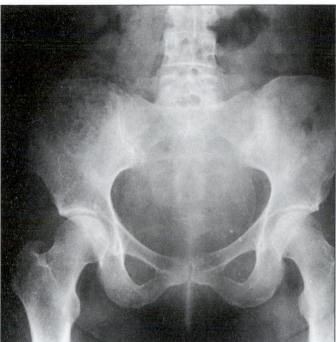

b

**Figure 5.109**

A 37-year-old woman with sacroiliitis. **(a)** Bone scan view of posterior pelvis; **(b)** X-ray of pelvis. Sacroiliac quantitation: left SIJ index 142, right SIJ index 148 (normal range 105–136). Both of these results are elevated and support the diagnosis of active sacroiliitis, which is confirmed on the X-ray.

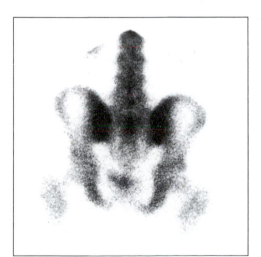

**Figure 5.110**

A 27-year-old man with sacroiliitis. Sacroiliac quantitation: left SIJ index 149, right SIJ index 144 (normal range 105–136).

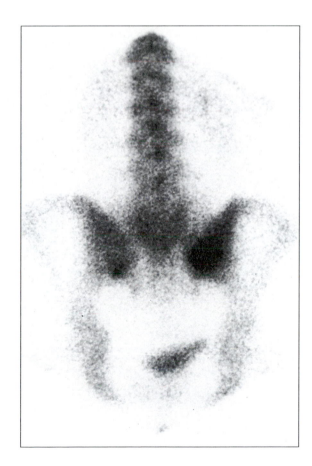

**Figure 5.111**

A 41-year-old woman with Crohn's disease and unilateral sacroiliitis. The right sacroiliac joint shows increased tracer uptake relative to the left. Sacroiliac quantitation: right SIJ index 144, left SIJ index 110 (normal range 105–136).

**Figure 5.112**

A 50-year-old woman with low back pain. Increased tracer uptake in the right sacroiliac joint (arrow) is appreciated on coronal SPECT **(a)** but not posterior view planar **(b)** bone scans. This patient was subsequently shown to have sacroiliitis.

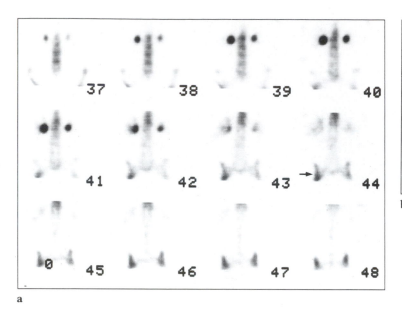

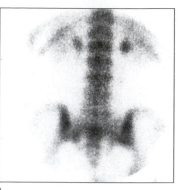

a

b

# Psoriatic arthropathy

**Figure 5.113**

**(a)** Bone scan of feet; **(b)** X-ray of left heel. The bone scan shows increased tracer uptake at the sites of insertion of the Achilles tendon and plantar fascia. The calcaneal changes are more marked on the left than on the right. The X-ray shows an erosion on the posterior aspect of the left calcaneus, with some overlying soft tissue thickening. This patient has psoriatic arthropathy with left-sided sacroiliitis, in addition to the calcaneal changes.

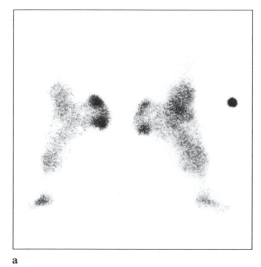

a

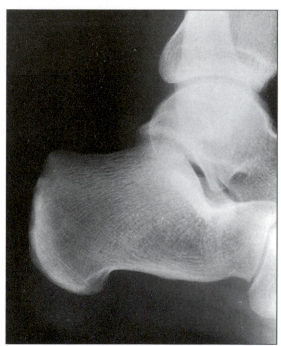

b

# Ankylosing spondylitis

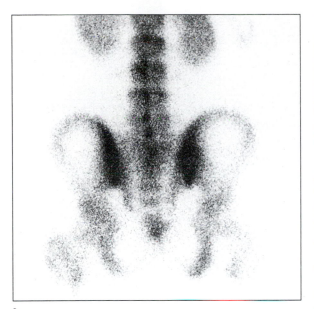

a

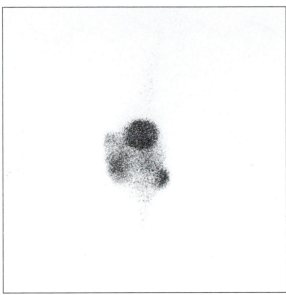

b

c

**Figure 5.114**

A 21-year-old man with ankylosing spondylitis. Bone scan views: **(a)** posterior pelvis, **(b)** left knee and **(c)** feet. Quantitation of the sacroiliac joint image revealed bilaterally high values. There is, in addition, abnormal tracer accumulation in the left knee, both ankles, os calcis and the right forefoot. There is also evidence of peripheral arthropathy.

**Figure 5.115**

A 47-year-old man with known ankylosing spondylitis. Planar bone scan views **(a, b)**, transaxial SPECT **(c)**, and coronal SPECT **(d)** of the thoracolumbar spine. There is increased tracer uptake in the region of the articular facets throughout much of the thoraco-lumbar spine. X-ray studies were normal.

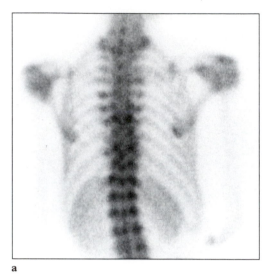

a

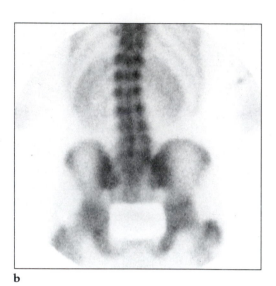

b

c

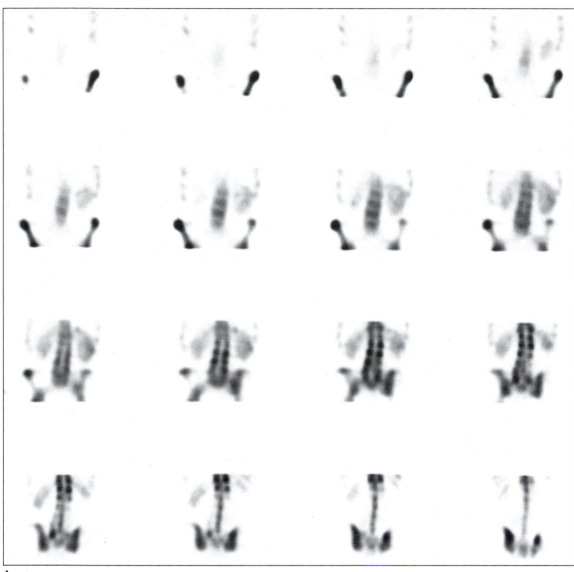

d

# Temporomandibular joint

**Figure 5.116**

A 25-year-old woman with 6 months of right TMJ pain, crepitus and limited opening. Anterior **(a)** and right lateral **(b)** planar bone scans suggest increased activity in the right TMJ, which is better localized on the transaxial SPECT image **(c)** (arrows). Magnetic resonance imaging confirmed internal derangement of the TMJ **(d)**

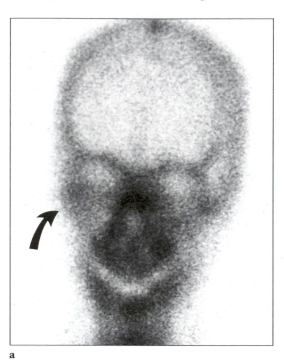

a

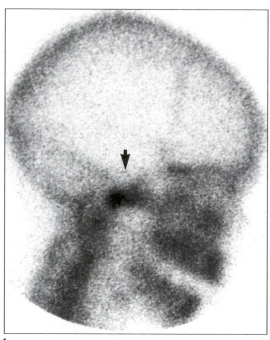

b

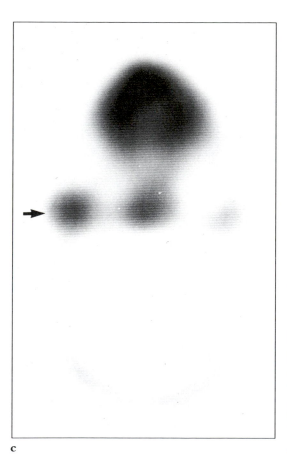

c

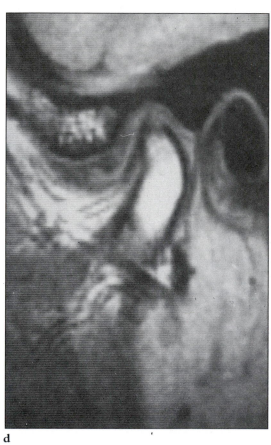

d

# Pigmented villonodular synovitis

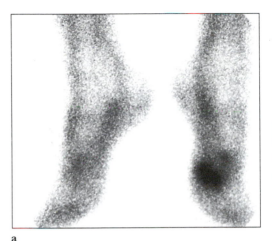

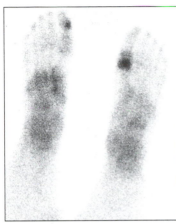

a b

**Figure 5.117**

A 44-year-old man who suffered for over 1 year from a painful enlargement of the left great toe. The anterior blood pool image (a) and plantar bone scan (b) show increased vascularity and tracer uptake at the left first MTP. The CT scan (c) shows a soft tissue mass in addition to bony erosions which have thin sclerotic margins. Biopsy established the diagnosis of pigmented villonodular synovitis.

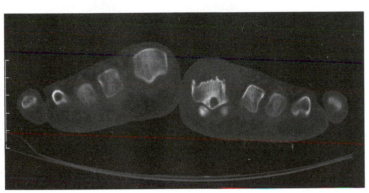

c

# Metabolic bone disease and other osteopathies

## Table 5.2 Bone scan in metabolic bone disease (MBD)

| Disease | Cause +ve bone scan | Differentiating features | Comment |
|---|---|---|---|
| Renal osteodystrophy | Hyperparathyroidism | Metabolic features<br>Absence of tracer in bladder | May find the most dramatic images seen in MBD |
| Primary hyperparathyroidism | Hyperparathyroidism | Metabolic features<br>Uncommon:<br>  brown tumours<br>  ectopic calcification | Bone scan usually normal |
| Osteomalacia | Hyperparathyroidism<br>Uptake in osteoid | Metabolic features<br>Pseudofractures (PF) | May not be possible to differentiate PF and metastases |
| Aluminium (Al)-induced osteomalacia | — | Low bone uptake<br>High background activity | Al is a bone poison which blocks mineralization |
| Osteoporosis | Fracture | Intense linear uptake at site of vertebral fracture<br>May be low/patchy uptake in axial skeleton | Bone scan usually normal<br>When there is fracture the bone scan cannot differentiate other causes, eg, tumour, on basis of scan alone<br>Activity at site of fracture fades over subsequent 1–2 years |

## Individual metabolic features

**Figure 5.118**

Increased tracer uptake throughout the calvaria and mandible.

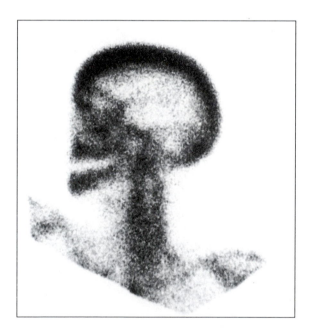

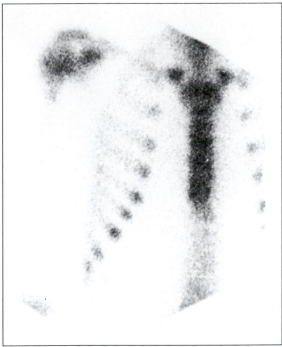

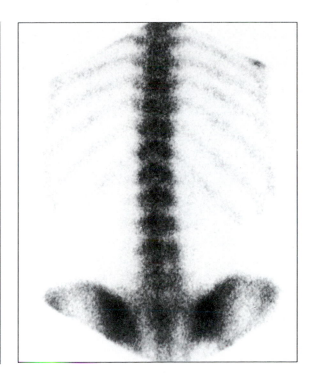

**Figure 5.119**

Increased tracer uptake at costochondral junctions (beading).

**Figure 5.120**

Increased uptake of tracer in the axial skeleton with high contrast between bone and soft tissue. The kidneys are not visualized.

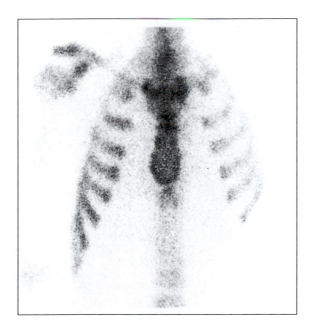

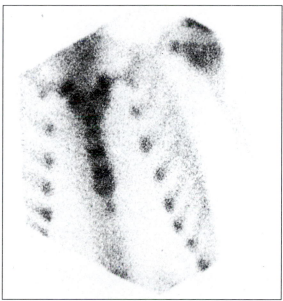

**Figure 5.121**

Increased tracer uptake throughout the sternum, the so-called tie sign.

**Figure 5.122**

Striped tie sign.

# Renal osteodystrophy

**Figure 5.123 (a–h)**

A 45-year-old woman with chronic renal failure. There is markedly increased tracer uptake throughout the whole skeleton and strikingly increased uptake in the calvaria and mandible; these appearances are typical of hyperparathyroidism. In addition, the renal images are not visualized. The scan findings are typical of metabolic bone disease and, in this case, represent severe renal osteodystrophy. Note that there is no activity present in the bladder.

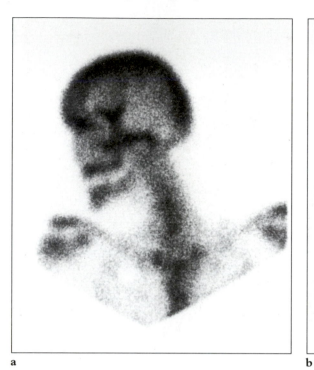

a

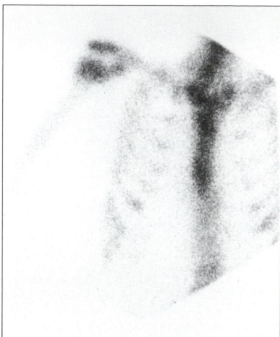

b

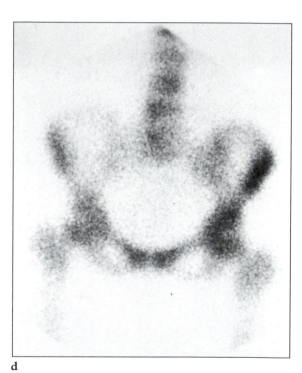

c

d

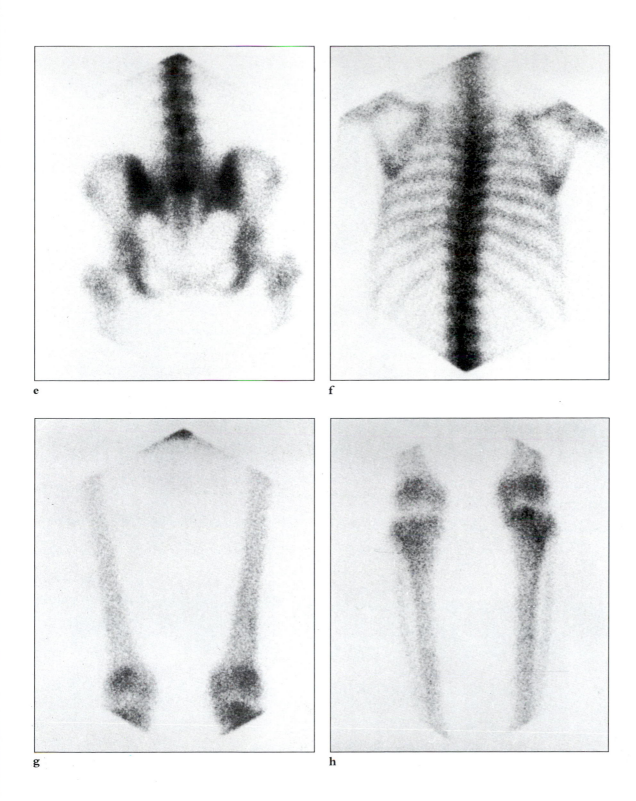

e

f

g

h

# Osteomalacia

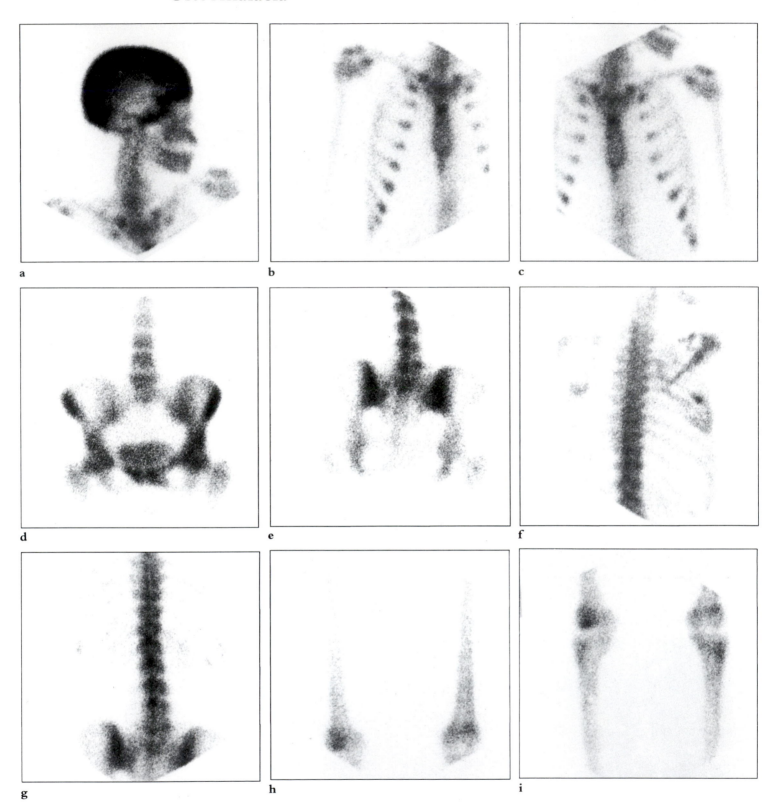

**Figure 5.124 (a–i)**

An Asian woman with osteomalacia. There is high uptake of tracer throughout the skeleton with several metabolic features present. In addition, there is a focal lesion in the right 4th rib posteriorly caused by a pseudofracture.

## Resolution of metabolic features

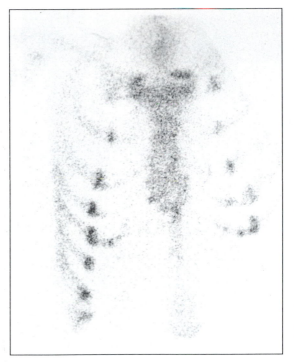

a

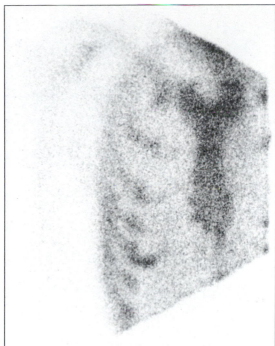

b

**Figure 5.125**
Bone scan views of anterior chest: **(a)** original study and **(b)** following surgery 2 months later. At the time of the original study, the patient had active acromegaly and increased tracer uptake is seen at the costochondral junctions. Following the transphenoidal removal of a pituitary tumour, the scan appearances are essentially normal, with a clear reduction in the avidity of the tracer uptake at the costochondral junctions.

## ■ Teaching point

■
Metabolic features are non-specific, but are often seen where there is increased skeletal metabolism, from whatever cause.

# Brown tumour in primary hyperparathyroidism

**Figure 5.126**

**(a)** Bone scan view of anterior tibiae; **(b)** X-ray of right tibia. Focal areas of increased tracer uptake are present in both upper tibiae caused by brown tumours, which are shown on the X-ray.

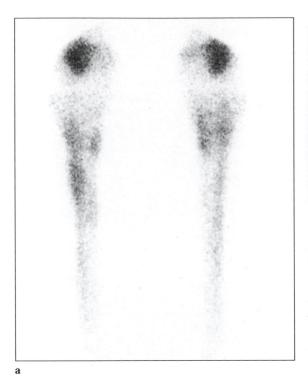

a

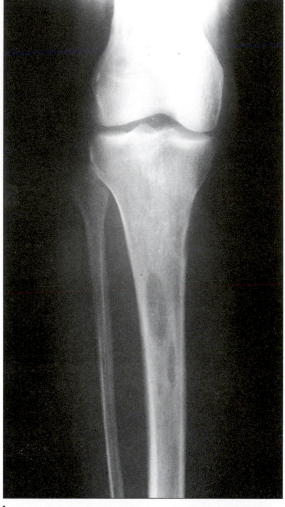

b

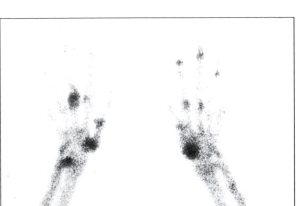

a

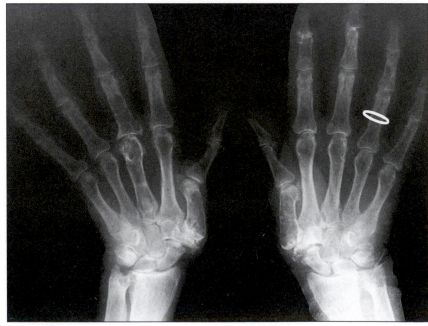

b

**Figure 5.127**

A further case of brown tumours involving the hands: **(a)** bone scan; **(b)** X-ray.

## Ectopic calcification related to hypercalcaemia

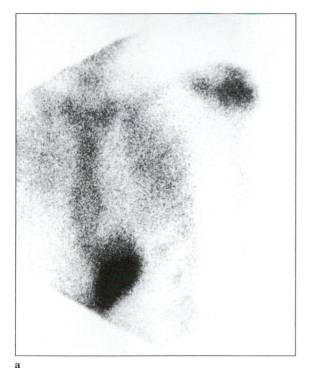

a

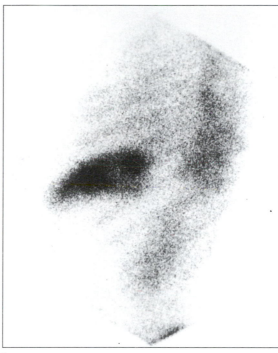

b

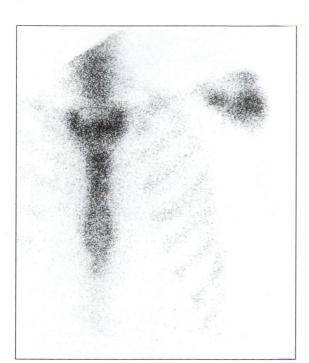

c

**Figure 5.128**

A 57-year-old man with severe hypercalcaemia caused by milk–alkali syndrome. Bone scan views: **(a)** anterior chest, **(b)** left lateral chest and **(c)** anterior chest 1 month later. This patient presented in acute renal failure, and serum calcium was found to be significantly elevated at 4 mmol/litre. The initial bone scan study shows strikingly increased tracer uptake in the stomach and lungs which is presumably related to microcalcification in these organs. Following rehydration and dialysis, this patient made a good recovery. The subsequent bone scan **(c)** is normal.

## ■ Teaching point

■ Scan features of ectopic calcification may be reversible in the short term.

# Pseudofractures

**Figure 5.129**

A 50-year-old Asian woman with osteomalacia who complained of pain in her ribs and difficulty in walking. Bone scan views: **(a)** posterior spine and thoracic cage and **(b)** pelvis and femora. The bone scans show multiple focal lesions in the ribs, pubic rami, left upper femur and neck of the right femur. There is generally high uptake of tracer throughout the skeleton and the renal images are not visualized, in keeping with metabolic bone disease. Focal lesions in this case represent pseudofractures.

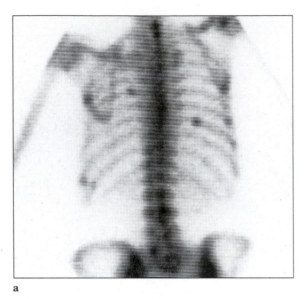

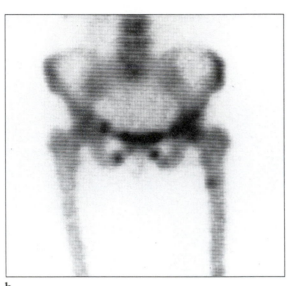

a

b

# Aluminium-induced bone disease

**Figure 5.130**

Bone scan views of posterior thoracic spine: **(a)** original study and **(b)** following desferrioxamine therapy. On the original study, there is very high background activity with poor delineation of bone. These findings are accounted for in this patient with chronic renal failure by aluminium-induced osteomalacia, where aluminium acts as a bone poison blocking mineralization. There is a dramatic improvement in the quality of the bone scan image following therapy.

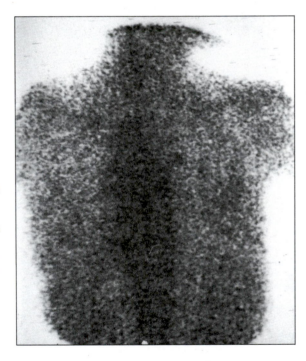

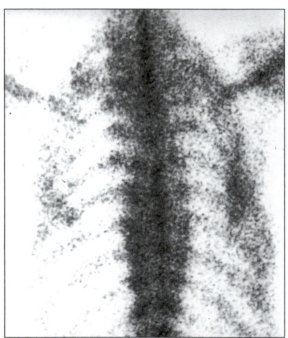

# Vertebral collapse associated with osteoporosis

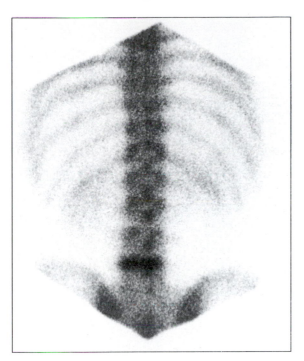

**Figure 5.131**

There is intense linearly increased tracer uptake in the region of L4. The scan appearances are typical of benign vertebral collapse, but the presence of coexistent pathology cannot be excluded.

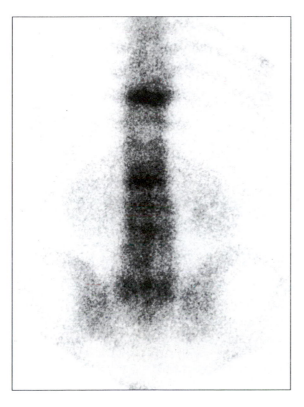

**Figure 5.132**

There are several areas of increased tracer uptake present at T10, L1 and L5, with non-homogeneity of tracer uptake throughout the remainder of the spine. Such scan appearances are often seen in patients with severe osteoporosis with multiple collapsed vertebrae.

## Resolution of osteoporotic collapse

**Figure 5.133**

An 82-year-old woman who experienced a sudden onset of severe back pain. Bone scan views of the posterior thoracic spine: **(a)** original study and **(b)** 8 months later; **(c)** lateral X-ray of spine. On the original study, there is markedly increased tracer uptake in a linear pattern associated with the collapsed vertebra seen on the X-ray at T8. On the repeat study, the abnormality is largely resolved. More often, a longer interval of 1–2 years is required before there is scan resolution in this situation.

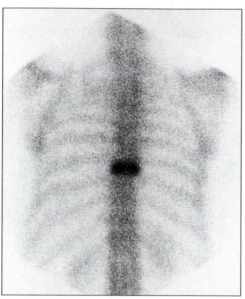

a

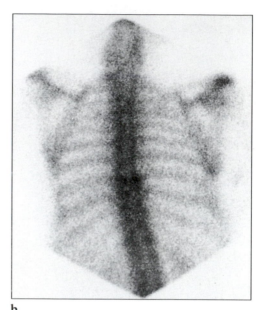

b

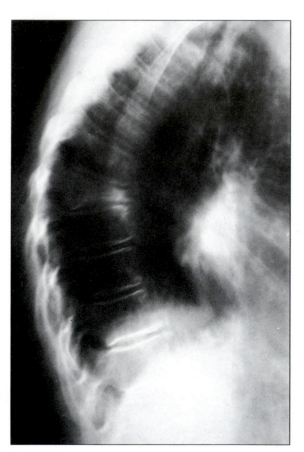

c

### ■ Teaching point

■
The bone scan may be of value in patients with known osteoporotic collapse in assessing the time interval since collapse occurred.

# Fluoride therapy

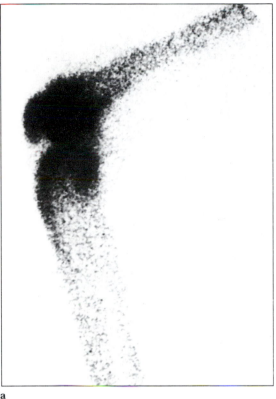

a

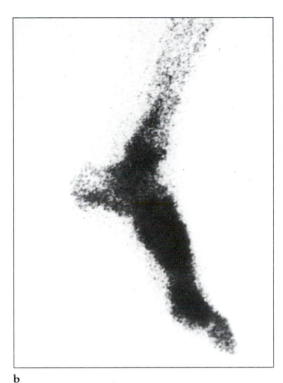

b

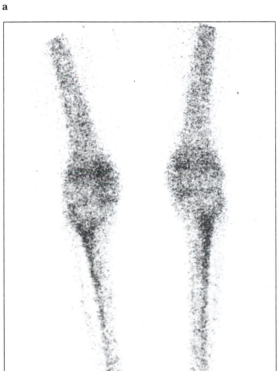

c

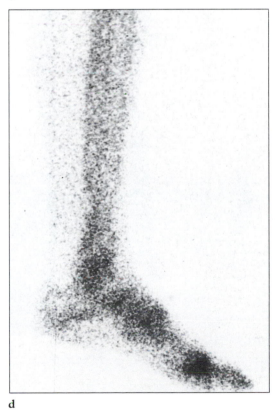

d

**Figure 5.134**

Bone scan views: **(a)** knee, **(b)** foot and **(c, d)** repeat 15 months later. This osteoporotic woman received fluoride therapy for 6 months and developed pain in her lower limbs. The scan **(a, b)** shows increased tracer uptake in multiple bones in the knee, ankle and foot. Therapy was discontinued, symptoms resolved, and the repeat study is essentially normal.

## Comment

■ There is some controversy as to the mechanism of acute lower extremity pain in fluoride-treated patients. Some reports have suggested that this is due to microfractures; others to a periosteal reaction.

# Thyroid acropachy

**Figure 5.135**

(a) Bone scan view of hands, (b) X-ray of hands, (c) bone scan view of tibiae and (d) X-ray of tibiae. The bone scan in thyrotoxicosis is most often normal but, depending on the severity of disease, may show metabolic features. In this patient with severe Graves' disease, increased patchy tracer accumulation is present in both hands, with more markedly increased uptake seen in the mid-tibiae. The scan findings are in keeping with the X-ray changes of thyroid acropachy, an uncommon complication of this disease. The patient also had severe eye disease and pretibial myxoedema.

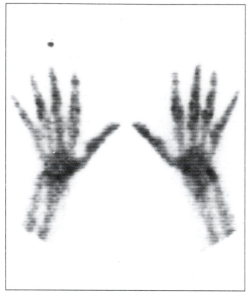

a

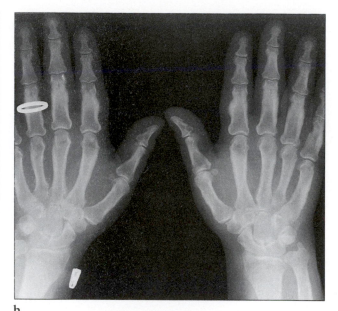

b

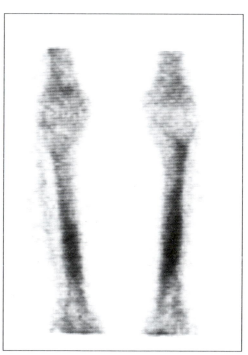

c

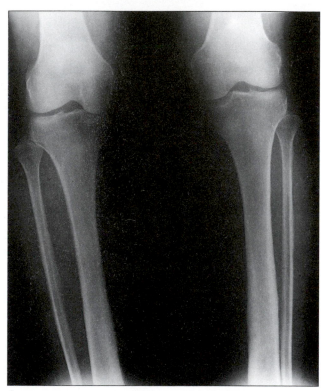

d

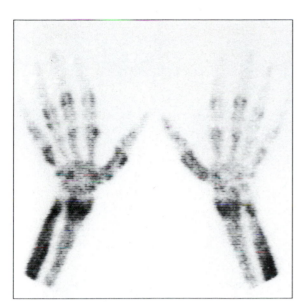

**Figure 5.136**

A striking case of thyroid acropachy involving the forearms and hands.

## Melorheostosis

**Figure 5.137**

(a) Bone scan view of femora; (b) X-ray of left femur. There is increased tracer uptake in the left femur associated with the lateral cortical border. This corresponds to changes seen on the X-ray, which are typically those of melorheostosis.

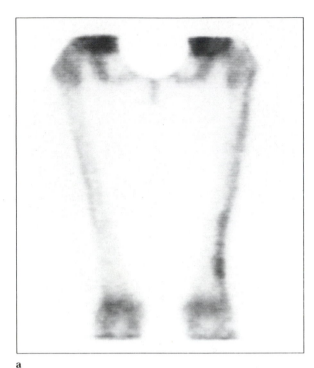

a

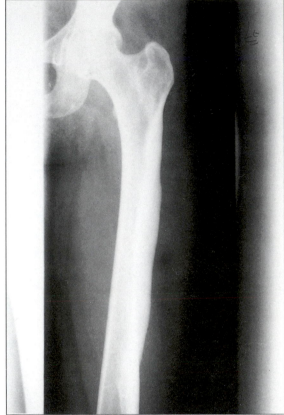

b

# Osteopoikilosis

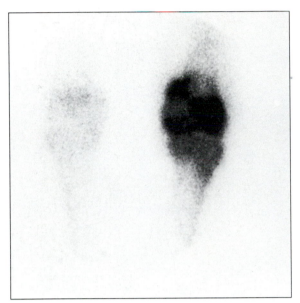

a

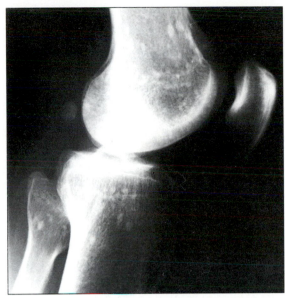

b

**Figure 5.138**

A 90-year-old man who presented with pain in his left knee due to a tumour. Bone scan view of **(a)** anterior knees; **(b)** X-ray of lateral right knee. There is intense increased tracer uptake associated with the tumour in the left knee. However, the right knee appears normal. The X-ray of the knee showed osteopoikilosis as an incidental finding. While there is little experience of bone scanning in this disorder, both osteopoikilosis and osteopathia striata are usually normal.

# Engelmann's disease

**Figure 5.139**

Bone scan views: **(a)** right lateral skull, **(b)** right anterior chest, **(c)** posterior thoracic spine, **(d)** left anterior chest, **(e)** anterior pelvis, **(f)** anterior femora, **(g)** anterior tibiae and **(h)** forearms. X-rays: **(i)** pelvis, **(j)** tibia and **(k)** forearm. There is increased patchy tracer uptake throughout the diaphyseal areas of all long bones, and also throughout the skull and the 11th rib posteriorly. Scan findings were due to Engelmann's disease, as shown on the X-ray.

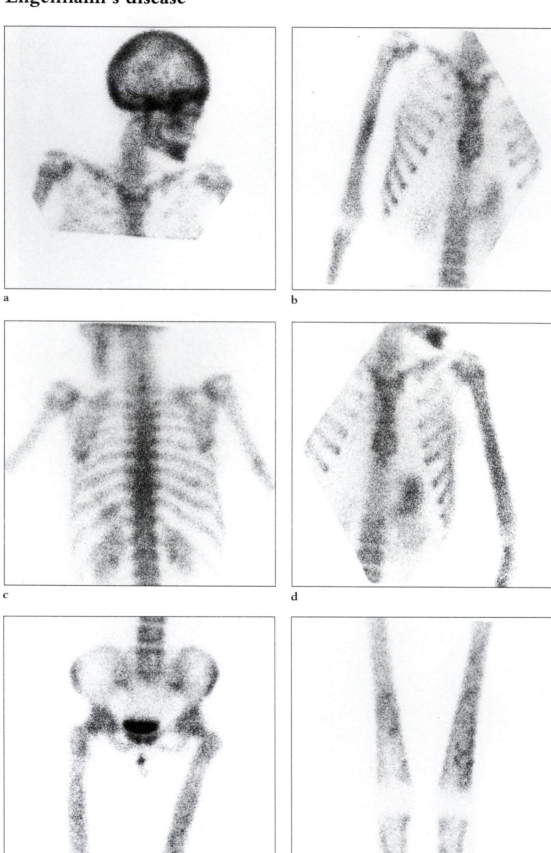

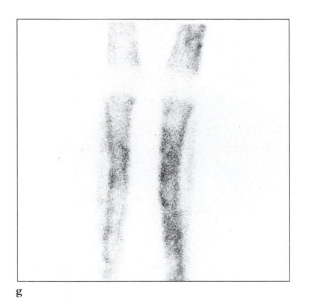

g

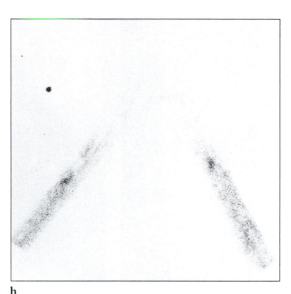

h

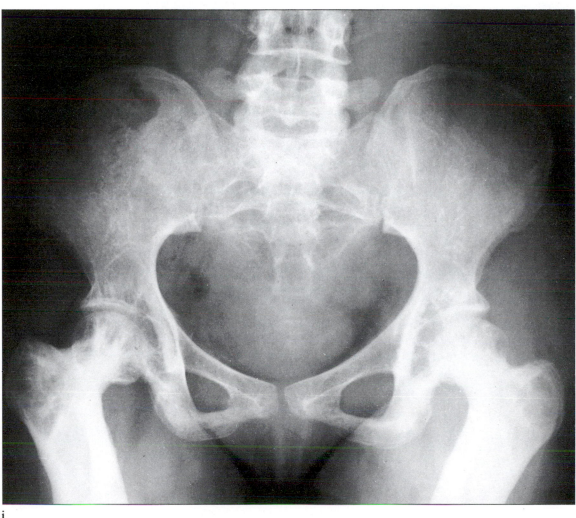

i

**Figure 5.139** *continued*

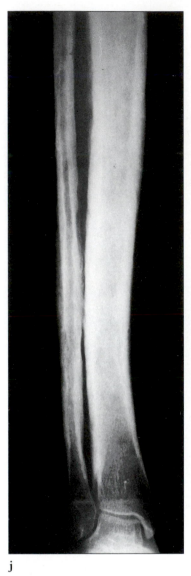

j

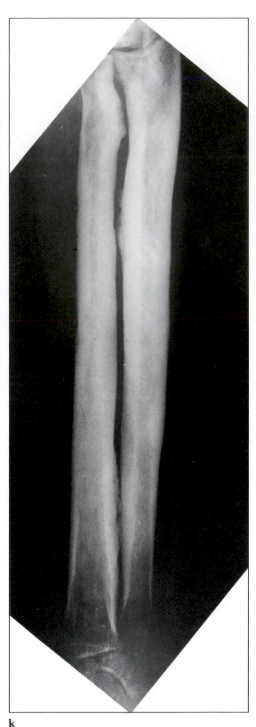

k

## Fibrous dysplasia

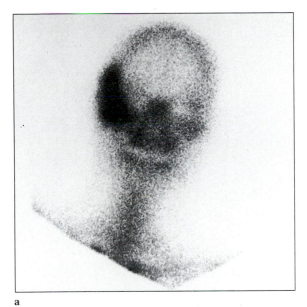

a

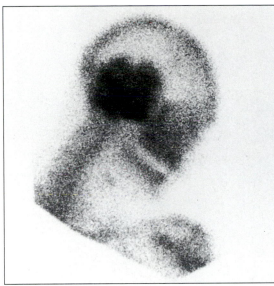

b

**Figure 5.140**

A 17-year-old boy who presented with deafness. Bone scan views: **(a)** anterior, **(b)** right lateral skull and **(c)** CT skull. There is massive abnormal tracer accumulation associated with the right temporal bone. The CT scan shows bony thickening typical of fibrous dysplasia, and note that there is occlusion of the auditory canal. Histological confirmation of diagnosis was established in this case.

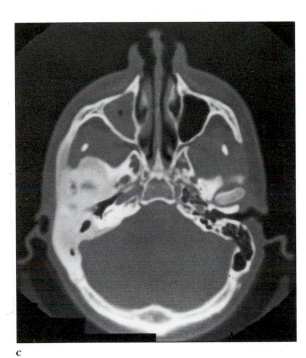

c

## ■ Teaching point

■ Approximately 20 per cent of cases of fibrous dysplasia are monostotic.

**Figure 5.141**

A 35-year-old woman with extensive fibrous dysplasia. Bone scan views: **(a)** anterior, **(b)** left lateral, **(c)** posterior skull, **(d)** right anterior chest, **(e)** left anterior chest, **(f)** posterior thoracic spine, **(g)** posterior lumbar spine. X-rays: **(h)** anterior and **(i)** lateral skull, **(j)** right and **(k)** left humerus. There is strikingly increased tracer uptake throughout many ribs, mostly on the left, with further focal abnormalities present in the spine, left hemipelvis, both humeri and skull. Note the large lesion in the skull extending outside normal bony margins. X-rays confirm fibrous dysplasia.

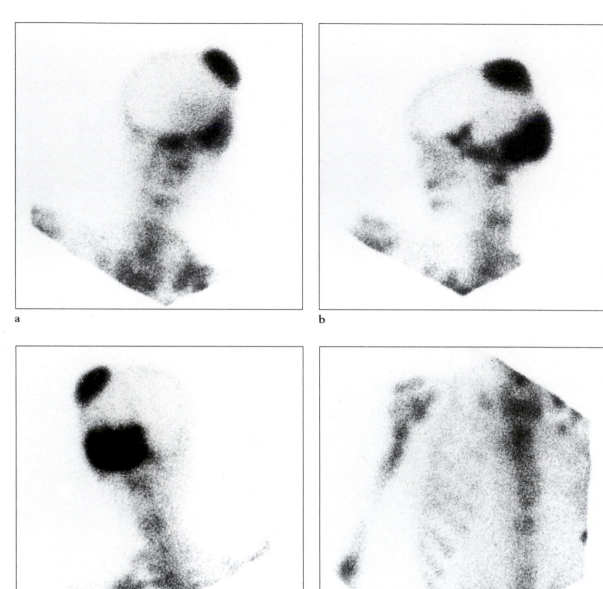

a

b

c

d

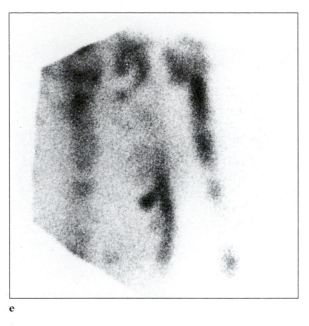

e

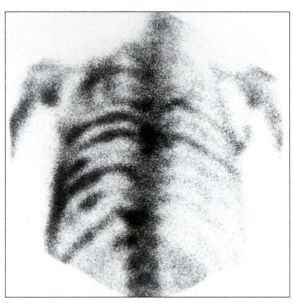

f

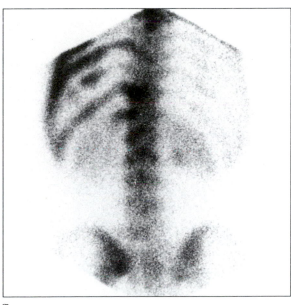

g

**Figure 5.141** *continued*

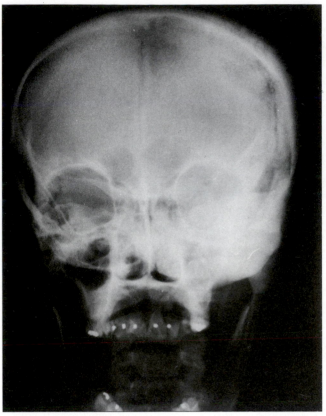

h

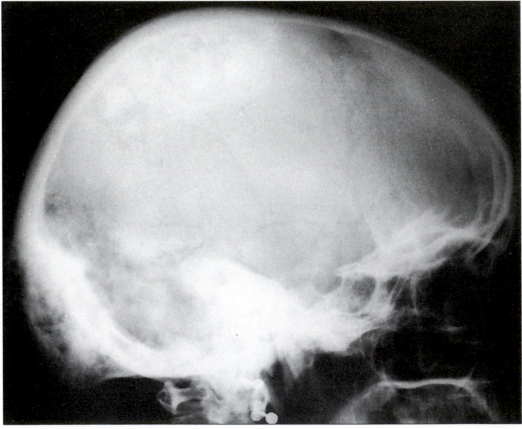

i

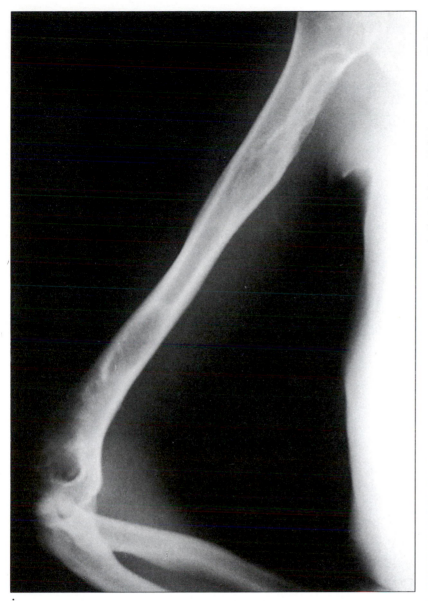

j

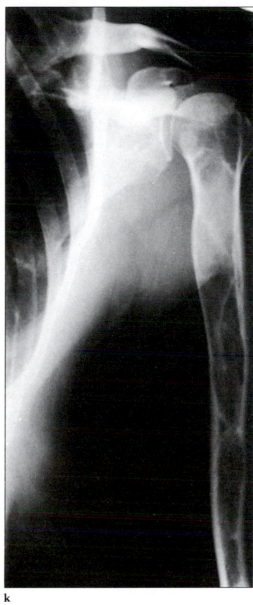

k

## ■ Teaching point

■
While lesions in polyostotic fibrous dysplasia are often unilateral, they may be bilateral as demonstrated in the above case.

# Paget's disease

■ **Bone scan features of Paget's disease:**

Intense uptake of tracer
Diffuse involvement of bone
Anatomical features may be emphasized,
  eg, transverse processes in spine
Ends of long bones affected, rather than
  diaphyseal disease
Expansion of bone
Deformity, eg, bowing of a long bone
Gradual change only over years
Polyostotic disease usually present
Spine and pelvis the most commonly
  involved sites

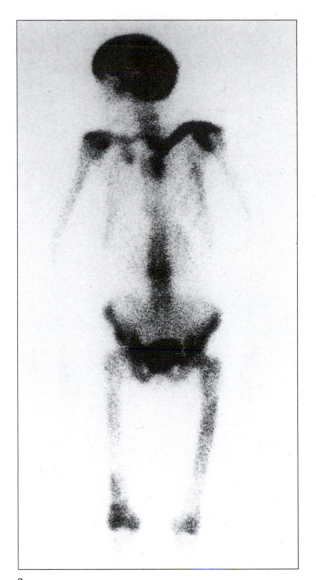

a

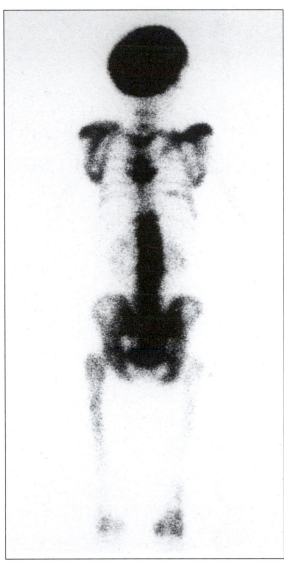

b

**Figure 5.142**

A 65-year-old woman with Paget's disease. Bone scan views: **(a)** anterior and **(b)** posterior. There is increased tracer uptake seen throughout the skull, left clavicle, both scapulae, thoracic and lumbar spine, pelvis and both femora. The scan findings are typical of extensive Paget's disease.

**Figure 5.143 (a–e)**

A further case of polyostotic Paget's disease. There is increased tracer uptake in the left tibia, left hemipelvis, L5, T7, maxilla and left clavicle. The scan findings are typical of Paget's disease involving the above sites.

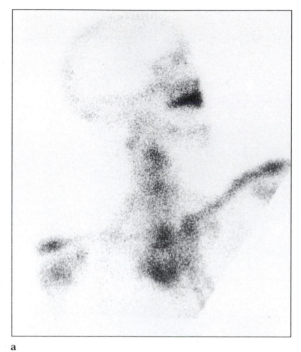

a

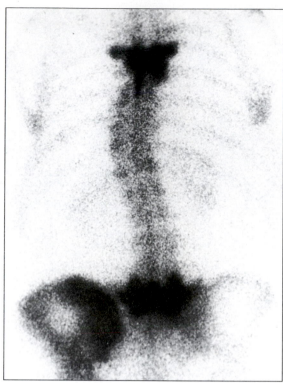

b

c

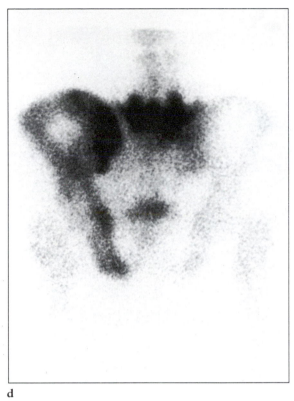

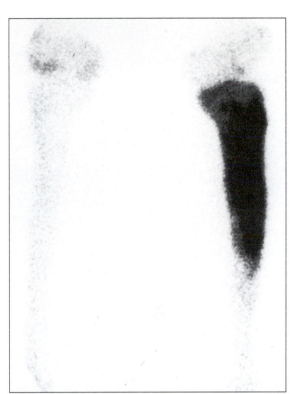

d                                        e

# Vascularity of pagetic bone

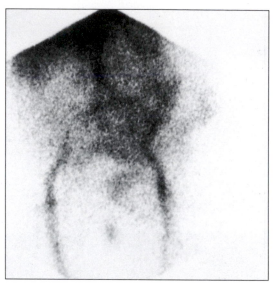

a

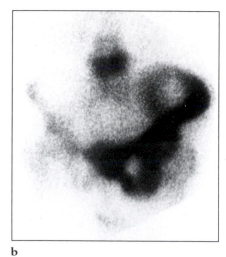

b

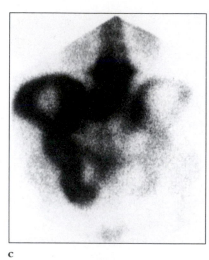

c

**Figure 5.144**

Bone scan views: **(a)** dynamic and **(b)** delayed images of anterior pelvis and **(c)** posterior pelvis; **(d)** X-ray of pelvis. There is strikingly increased tracer uptake throughout the whole of the left hemipelvis and throughout the body of L5. The left hemipelvis is intensely vascular on the dynamic study. The scan appearances are typical of Paget's disease; this is confirmed on the X-ray.

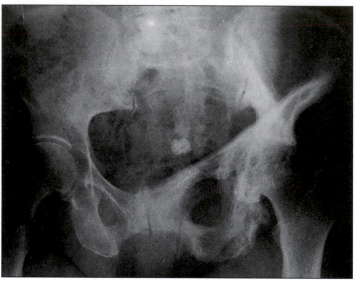

d

## Monostotic Paget's disease

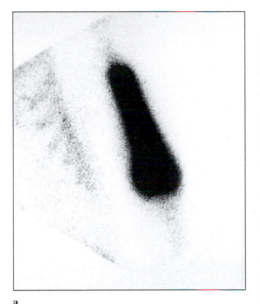

a

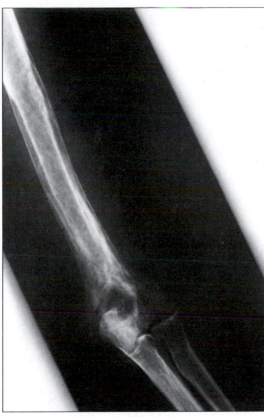

b

**Figure 5.145**

An 84-year-old man with monostotic Paget's disease involving the left humerus. **(a)** Bone scan view of left chest and humerus; **(b)** X-ray of left humerus. On the bone scan image there is strikingly increased tracer uptake throughout the left lower humerus. The scan appearances are typical of Paget's disease; this is confirmed on the X-ray.

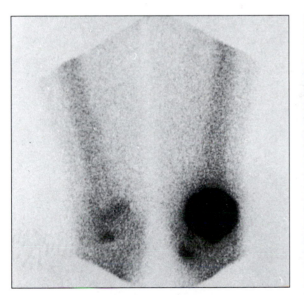

a

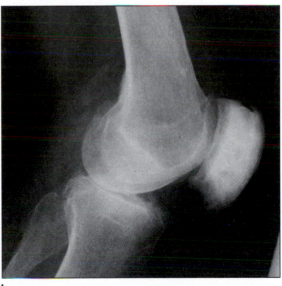

b

**Figure 5.146**

A 75-year-old man with monostotic Paget's disease involving the patella. **(a)** Bone scan view of anterior lower femora and knees; **(b)** X-ray of lateral left knee. The bone scan image shows strikingly increased tracer uptake throughout the left patella. The X-ray confirms Paget's disease at this site. The bone scan is otherwise normal; thus this is a most unusual case of monostotic Paget's disease involving the left patella.

## ■ Teaching point

■
Monostotic Paget's disease is not uncommon and accounts for approximately 20 per cent of cases.

# Further examples of Paget's disease

**Figure 5.147 (a–c)**

Three cases of Paget's disease involving the skull.

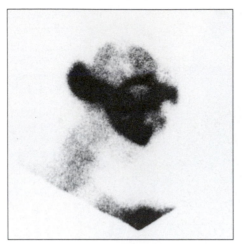

a

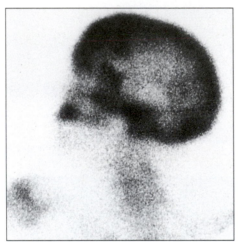

b

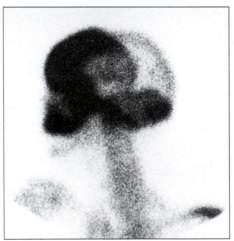

c

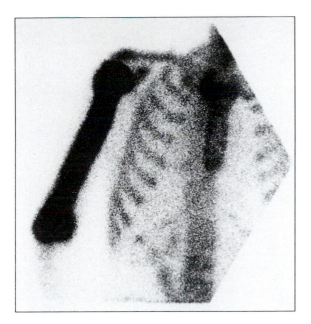

**Figure 5.148**

Paget's disease involving
the right humerus.

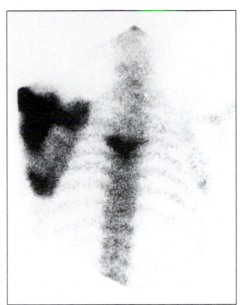

**Figure 5.149**

Paget's disease involving
the left scapula and T5.

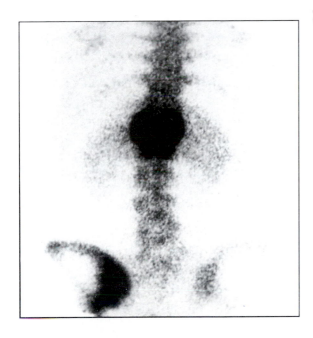

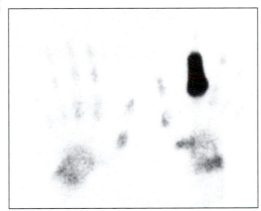

**Figure 5.151**

Paget's disease involving
the left 1st proximal
phalanx.

**Figure 5.150**

Paget's disease involving
L1 and the left hemipelvis.

# Progression of Paget's disease

**Figure 5.152**

On the original study **(a, b)** in 1977, the typical scan appearances of Paget's disease involving the left humerus and left hemipelvis are seen. Further scans taken in 1979 **(c, d)** and 1985 **(e, f)** show little change in these findings. However, the latter show involvement of the sacrum, which was not apparent in 1977. In the authors' experience, it is most unusual to be able to document the development and progression of Paget's disease.

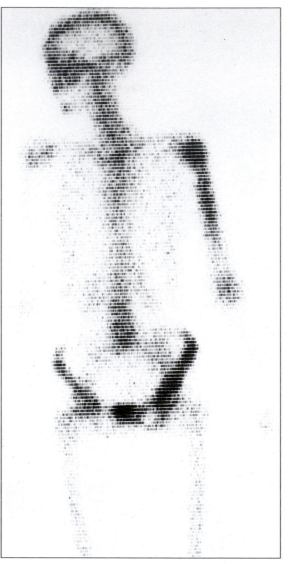

a

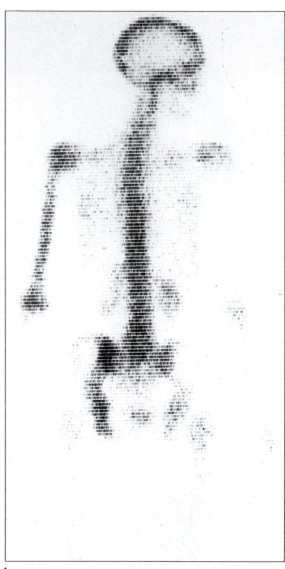

b

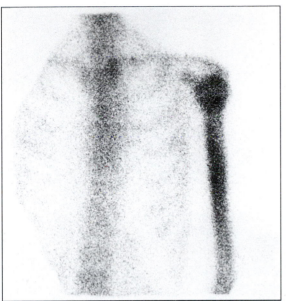

c

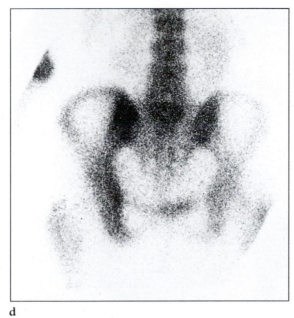

d

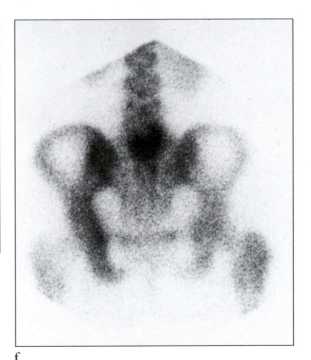

e

f

## ■ Teaching point

■ If changes occur in a bone scan over a relatively short period of time, they should not be attributed to Paget's disease, and other pathology should be considered.

# Response to therapy

**Figure 5.153**

A 63-year-old woman with Paget's disease. Bone scan views of the posterior pelvis and upper femora: **(a)** original study and **(b)** following therapy. There is markedly increased tracer uptake throughout the left hemipelvis and upper femur. These scan appearances are typical of Paget's disease. Following 9 months' treatment with oral diphosphonate, there has been striking resolution of disease.

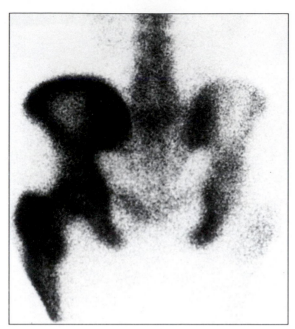

a

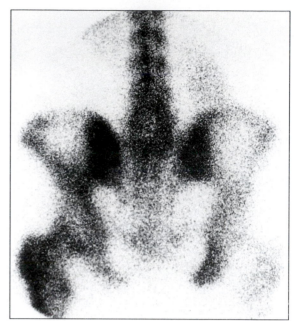

b

# Fracture

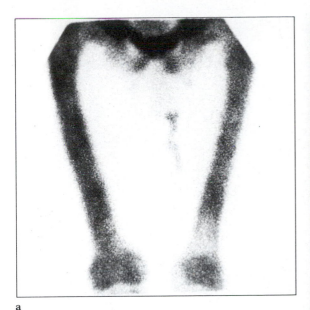

a

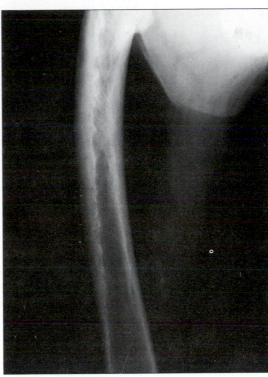

b

**Figure 5.154**

An elderly man with known extensive Paget's disease who complained of pain in his right leg. **(a)** Bone scan view of femora; **(b)** X-ray of right femur. On the bone scan, there is increased but patchy tracer uptake in both femora, which is most pronounced on the right. The X-ray reveals multiple stress fractures. Although the tracer uptake is patchy on the scan image, the degree of abnormality revealed on the X-ray was not suspected. Furthermore, there is patchy tracer uptake in the left femur, but the X-ray did not reveal fracture.

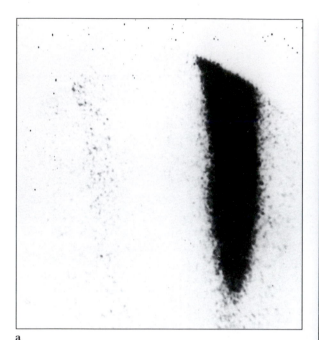

a

**Figure 5.155**

Paget's fracture. **(a)** Bone scan view of tibiae; **(b)** X-ray. There is intense uptake of tracer throughout the left tibia. Scan findings are typically those of Paget's disease. While the X-ray confirms the presence of Paget's disease there is, however, a fracture present. This is not apparent on the bone scan due to generalized high uptake of tracer throughout the whole of the pagetic bone.

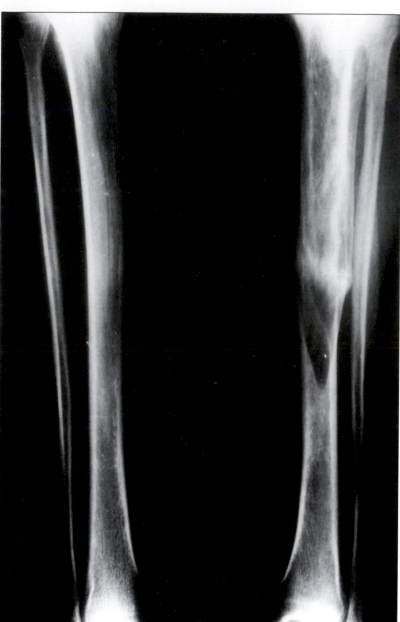

b

## ■ Teaching point

■ The bone scan is not adequate to exclude fracture in patients with Paget's disease. This is because increased tracer uptake associated with fracture may not be recognized against high background activity.

# Osteogenic sarcoma and Paget's disease

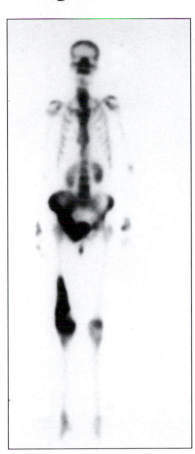

**Figure 5.156**

A patient with known Paget's disease of the pelvis and right femur who presented with pain in his right leg. The bone scan shows a focal defect at the medial aspect of the right lower tibia, and destructive changes were identified at this site by radiography. This patient had an osteogenic sarcoma associated with Paget's disease.

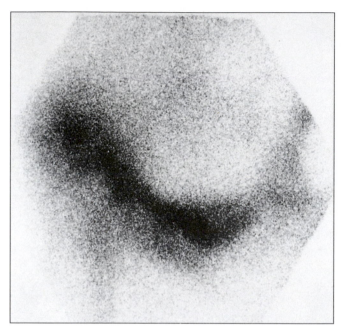
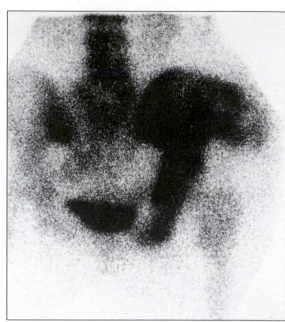

a

b

**Figure 5.157**

Bone scan views of pelvis: **(a)** anterior and **(b)** posterior; **(c)** X-ray of pelvis. The bone scans show extensive abnormal tracer accumulation throughout the right hemipelvis, with gross disruption of the anatomical borders in the lateral portion of the iliac wing. Note also that there is tracer uptake in associated soft tissue. The X-ray shows evidence of gross destruction at the corresponding site, together with the changes of Paget's disease. The scan appearances and X-ray findings are attributable to known Paget's disease, with the expanded destructive appearance caused by sarcomatous change.

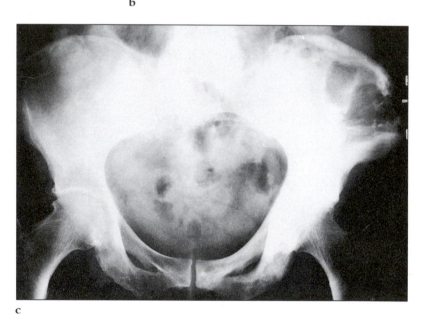

c

## ■ Teaching points

■

If sarcomatous change is suspected in a patient with known Paget's disease, radiographic investigation is required for evaluation, because, as with fracture, increased uptake may not always be apparent.

■

While sarcomatous change normally appears 'hot' on the bone scan, this is not always the case.

# Coexistent Paget's disease and metastatic disease

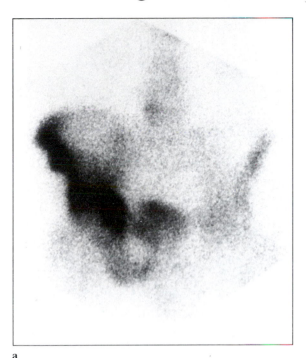

a

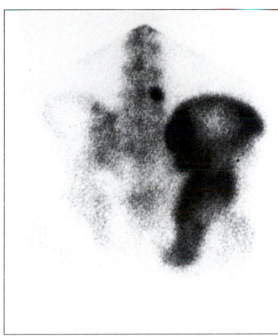

b

**Figure 5.158**

The bone scans **(a, b)** show the typical features of Paget's disease involving the right hemipelvis. In addition, however, multiple focal abnormalities are present in the spine and ribs which are typical of metastases **(c)**. The X-ray of the pelvis **(d)** confirms Paget's disease, while the X-ray of the spine **(e)** confirms the presence of metastases.

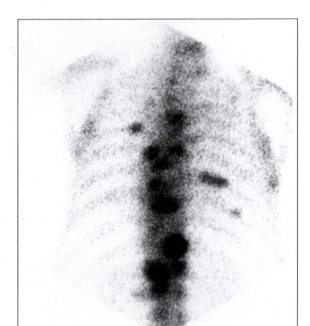

c

**Figure 5.158** *continued*

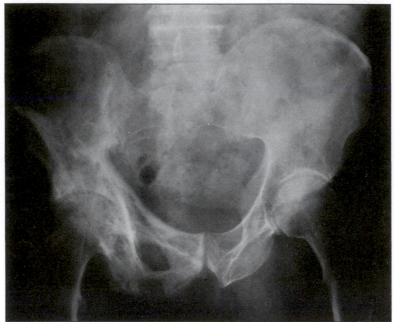

d

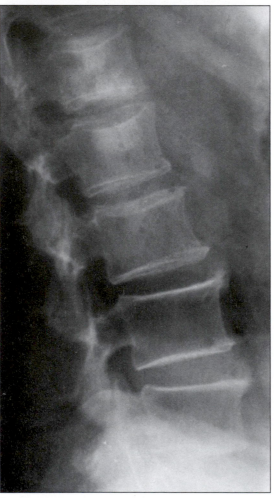

e

# ■ Teaching point

■ Although Paget's disease and metastases usually show characteristic scan patterns of abnormality and can be easily differentiated, radiographic examination is still required for confirmation, because on occasion, each of these conditions can mimic the other.

# Metabolic activity of a lesion

## Bone island

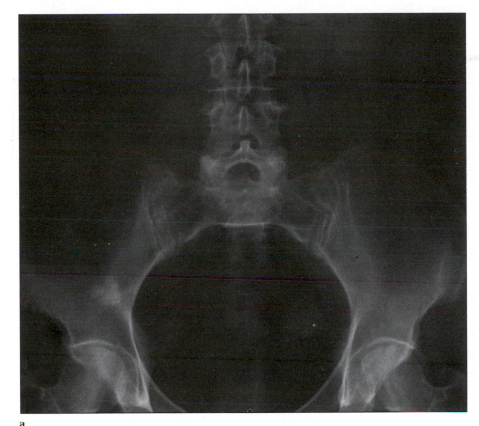

a

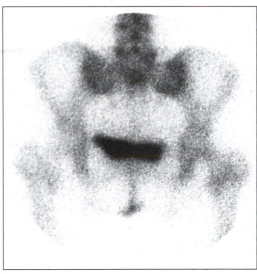

b

**Figure 5.159**

A 64-year-old woman with low back pain and a history of colonic carcinoma. The X-ray **(a)** shows a sclerotic lesion in the right ilium with an appearance typical of a bone island. However, in view of the symptoms and previous carcinoma a bone scan was obtained. The benign and metabolically inactive nature of this lesion is confirmed by the normal bone scan **(b)**.

## ■ Teaching point

■
While a bone island usually appears normal on a bone scan, this is not always the case.

# Chondroma

**Figure 5.160**

Chondroma of the rib. **(a)** Bone scan view of the anterior chest; **(b)** chest X-ray. This 25-year-old woman was noted to have a calcified lesion in her right 2nd rib on chest X-ray. It was thought to be a benign chondroma. A bone scan was requested to assess metabolic activity. It is apparent that the lesion is barely visible, with only faintly increased tracer uptake at that site. Scan appearances are in keeping with the benign nature of the lesion.

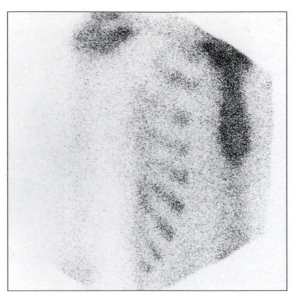

a

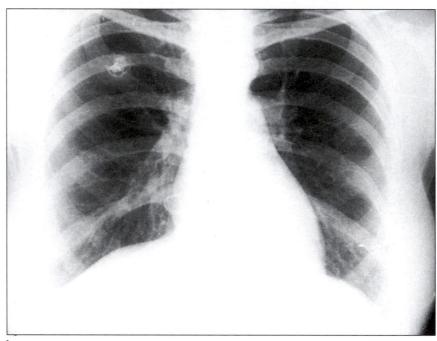

b

# Bone infarct

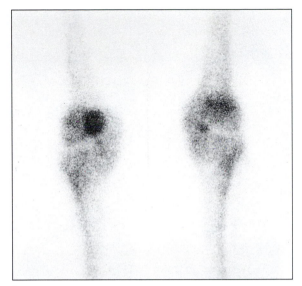

a

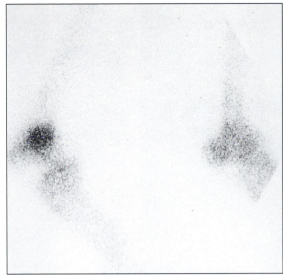

b

**Figure 5.161**
Bone scan views of knees:
**(a)** anterior and **(b)** right
medial; **(c)** X-ray of right
lateral knee. There is a
single area of increased
radionuclide accumulation
between the condyles of
the right femur which
corresponds to the
sclerotic lesion seen on the
X-ray. It was felt that the
lesion represented a bone
infarct. Note that on the
anterior view alone the
scan appearances could be
mistaken for the 'hot'
patella sign.

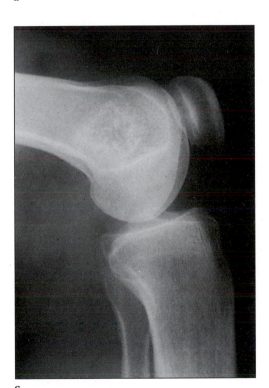

c

# Treated osteomyelitis

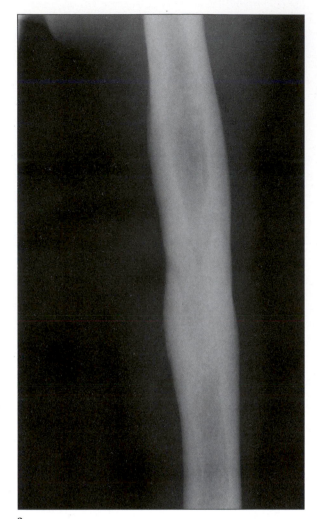

a

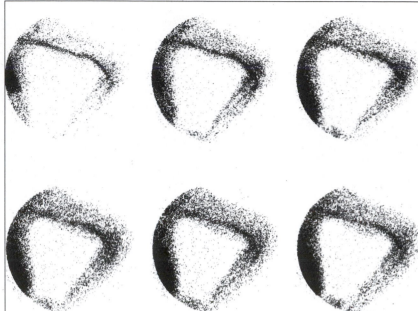

b

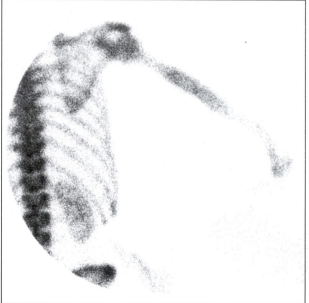

c

**Figure 5.162**

A 23-year-old man with a history of osteomyelitis treated 3 years previously, who was evaluated for possible recurrence in the right humerus. The X-ray **(a)** shows a thick periosteal reaction, a finding which neither confirms nor disproves the diagnosis of active osteomyelitis. Dynamic study **(b)** and posterior bone scan images of the right humerus **(c)** show normal vascularity along with slight prominence of uptake at the site of periosteal thickening. This can be accounted for by continuing bony remodelling. If active osteomyelitis were present, there would be much more intense tracer uptake.

# Miscellaneous topics    6

- Extraskeletal localization of diphosphonate
- Localization of lesion
- Thoracoplasty
- Rib resection
- Vascular abnormalities
- Urinary tract

## Extraskeletal localization of diphosphonate

There are many situations in which
diphosphonate may localize in soft tissues,
and the common factor for these appears to be
the presence of microcalcification.

## Diphosphonate uptake in cerebrovascular accident

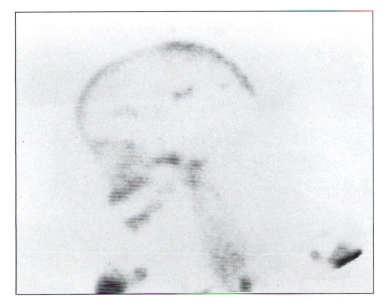

**Figure 6.1**

Bone scan view of
lateral skull showing three
foci of diphosphonate
accumulation in the
left hemisphere,
corresponding to a known
cerebral infarct.

# Pulmonary uptake

**Figure 6.2**

Lung uptake due to hypercalcaemia. Bone scan views: **(a)** left anterior chest; **(b)** same 6 months later. There is strikingly increased tracer uptake seen diffusely over lung fields, and note also the tracer in the stomach. This patient had severe hypercalcaemia related to carcinoma of the breast at that time. Hypercalcaemia was successfully treated, and the study 6 months later shows resolution of these abnormalities.

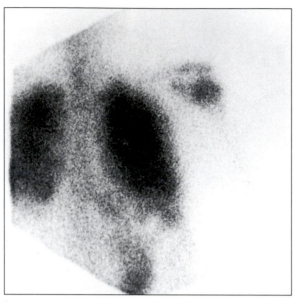

a

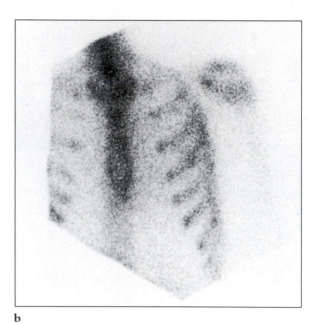

b

# Splenic infarct

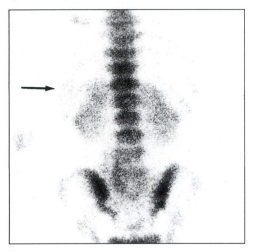

a

b

c

**Figure 6.3**

A case of sickle cell disease. **(a)** Bone scan view of posterior lumbar spine, **(b)** liver scan anterior view and **(c)** liver scan posterior view. On the bone scan, there is faint tracer uptake by the spleen (arrow). On the liver scan, the spleen is not visualized. This patient, therefore, has functional asplenia caused by previous splenic infarction.

# Repeated intramuscular injections

**Figure 6.4**

Bone scan views of pelvis: **(a)** anterior and **(b)** posterior. There is a large area of abnormal tracer uptake lateral to the right hip (arrows) which is caused by repeated intramuscular injections.

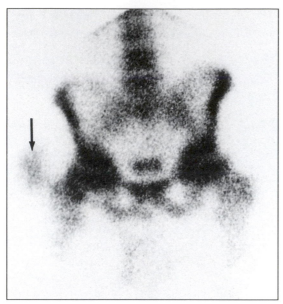

a

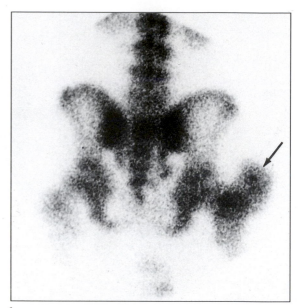

b

**Figure 6.5**

A 32-year-old man with severe back pain was given repeated injections of meperidine into the anterior aspect of both thighs. An anterior bone scan of the thighs shows soft tissue uptake of tracer within the injected muscles.

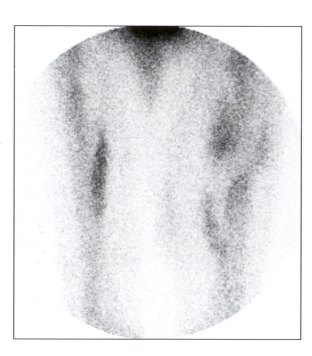

# Amyloid

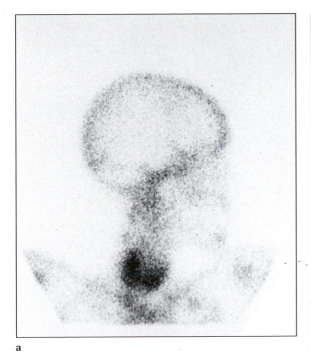

a

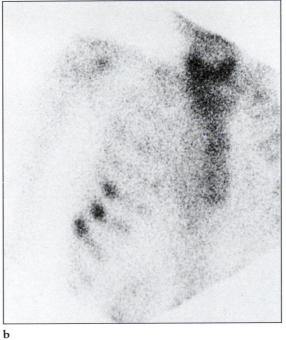

b

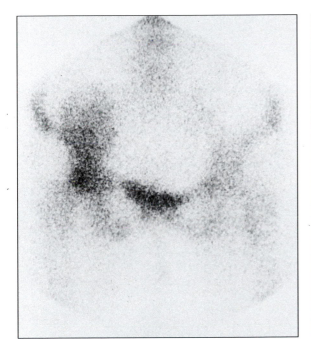

c

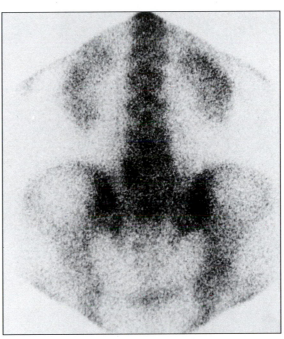

d

**Figure 6.6**

A 63-year-old woman with a renal transplant for amyloid kidney. Bone scan views: **(a)** right skull, **(b)** anterior chest, **(c)** anterior pelvis and **(d)** posterior lumbar spine and pelvis. Although this patient had a functioning renal transplant, which is seen in the right iliac fossa, tracer uptake is visualized in the host kidneys and there is also increased uptake present in the thyroid. There was no radiopharmaceutical problem, and the stomach was not visualized. These findings are due to uptake in the amyloid tissue. In addition, focal abnormalities are noted in the right anterior ribs caused by fracture following trauma. The uptake in the right femoral neck is accounted for by avascular necrosis.

# Muscle necrosis

**Figure 6.7**

A 34-year-old man who presented with acute renal failure secondary to rhabdomyolysis. Bone scan view: **(a)** left anterior chest, **(b)** anterior pelvis, **(c)** posterior pelvis and **(d–f)** corresponding views on repeat study 11 days later. On the original study, there is massive accumulation of tracer in muscle, particularly in the hip girdle muscle. On the repeat study, there is dramatic resolution of the scan appearances, although the background tracer activity is slightly increased.

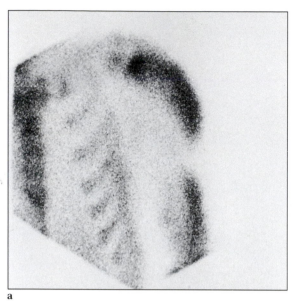

a

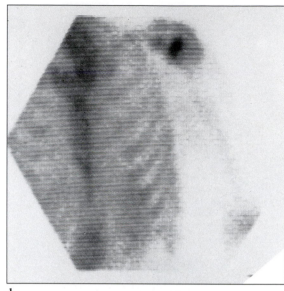

d

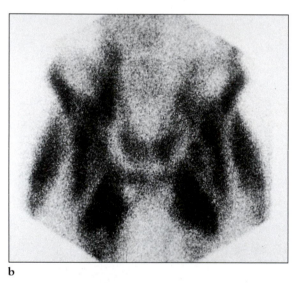

b

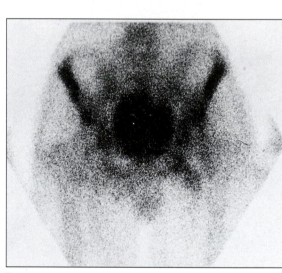

e

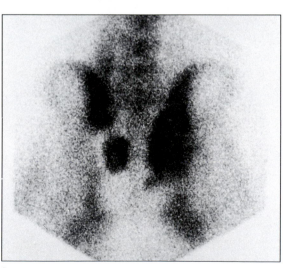

c

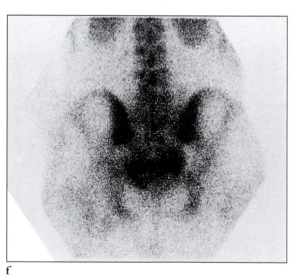

f

# Malignancy

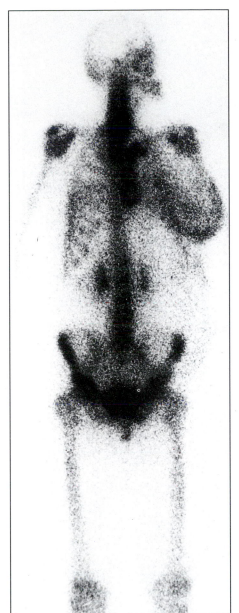

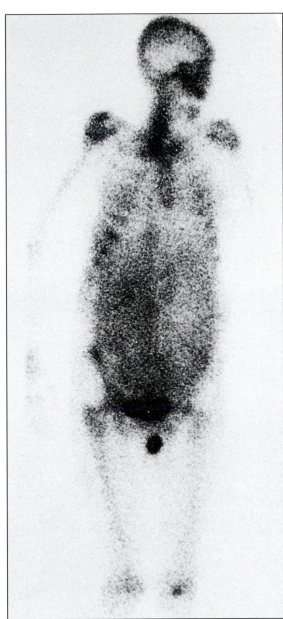

**Figure 6.8**

Breast. A patient with carcinoma of the left breast and associated 'peau-d'orange' changes.

**Figure 6.9**

Ascites. Increased tracer uptake is seen diffusely throughout the abdomen, related to known malignant ascites. No discrete focus is seen throughout the skeleton.

**Figure 6.10**

Pleural effusion. Bone scan views: **(a)** anterior chest, **(b)** posterior thorax; **(c)** X-ray of chest. The tracer uptake in the left hemithorax is related to a malignant pleural effusion, as seen on the X-ray. Also note focal abnormalities due to metastases in the sternum, the tip of the right scapula, and the left ribs anteriorly.

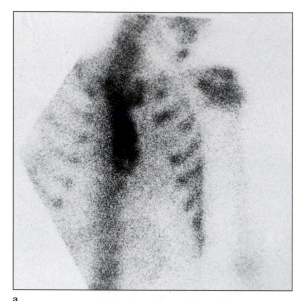

a

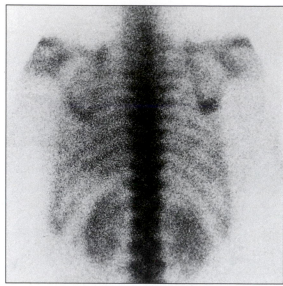

b

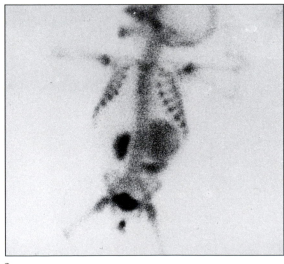

c

**Figure 6.11**

Tumour uptake in a neuroblastoma. Bone scan views: **(a)** anterior and **(b)** posterior. There is massive abnormal tracer accumulation associated with a left-sided adrenal tumour (neuroblastoma). Note that the left kidney is markedly rotated by the adrenal mass. No abnormality was present in the skeleton.

a

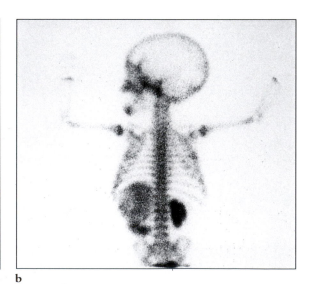

b

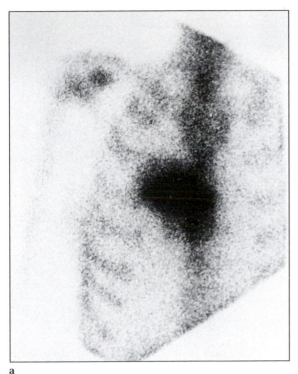

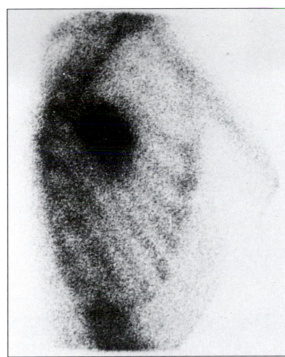

a

b

**Figure 6.12**

Tumour uptake. A 61-year-old woman with carcinoma of the oesophagus. Bone scan views of chest: **(a)** anterior and **(b)** right lateral. There is massive abnormal accumulation of tracer in the right posterior mediastinum. No focal abnormalities were seen in the skeleton. The tracer uptake in this case is associated with the primary oesophageal malignancy.

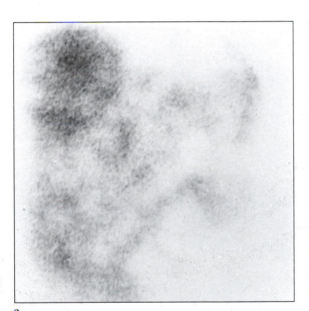

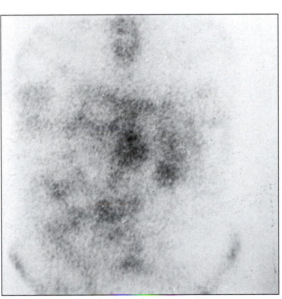

a

b

**Figure 6.13**

Uptake in metastases. **(a)** Liver scan and **(b)** bone scan view of anterior abdomen. This patient with medullary carcinoma of the thyroid had known hepatic metastases. The liver scan shows the liver to be markedly enlarged, with multiple focal defects throughout. On the bone scan image, there is tracer uptake in the liver, corresponding to the tumour.

**Figure 6.14**

Uptake in meningioma. Bone scan views of the skull: **(a)** left lateral and **(b)** anterior; **(c)** CT brain scan. On **(a)**, an intense focus of increased tracer uptake is seen. This patient was known to have carcinoma of the breast, and based on a lateral view alone, the physician would be justified to conclude that a skull lesion was present, most probably a metastasis. But **(b)** clearly shows that the lesion is intracerebral. A skull X-ray was not considered to be helpful, but the CT scan confirmed the presence of a meningioma. There were no other lesions in the skeleton.

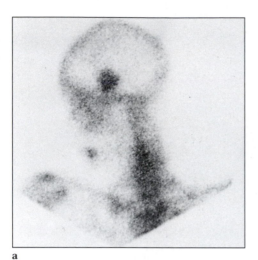

a

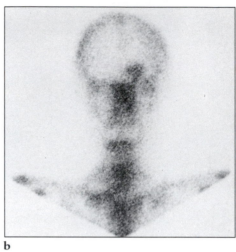

b

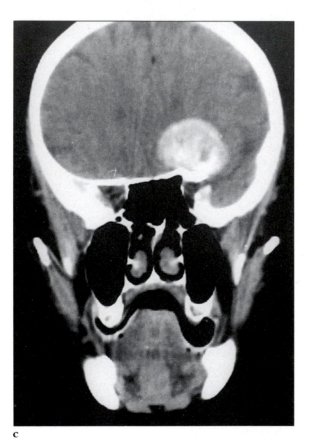

c

# Soft tissue calcification

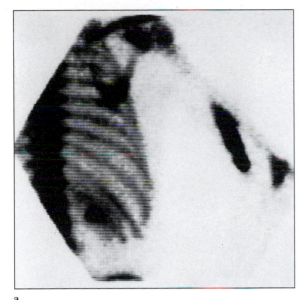

a

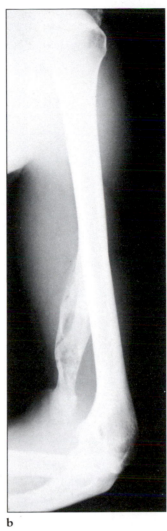

b

### Figure 6.15

A 22-year-old man with myositis ossificans.
**(a)** Bone scan of right posterior thorax and arm; **(b)** corresponding X-ray. There is increased tracer accumulation lying within the brachialis muscle, corresponding to the soft tissue calcification seen on the X-ray. The scan appearances represent continuing active bone turnover associated with myositis ossificans.

### Figure 6.16

A 71-year-old woman with ectopic calcification. **(a)** Bone scan view of anterior pelvis; **(b)** X-ray of pelvis. There is markedly increased tracer accumulation in the region of the greater trochanter and extending upwards, which is more pronounced on the right. This patient had severe renal bone disease with ectopic calcification, which is obvious on the X-ray. The patient also had avascular necrosis in both hips.

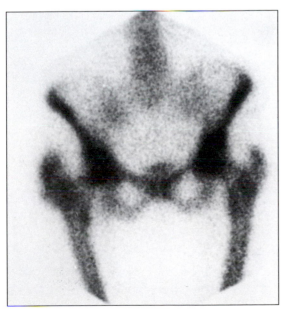

a

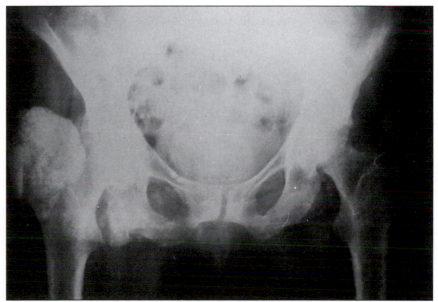

b

**Figure 6.17**

Bone scan **(a)** and X-ray **(b)** of hands in a patient with systemic sclerosis and calcinosis.

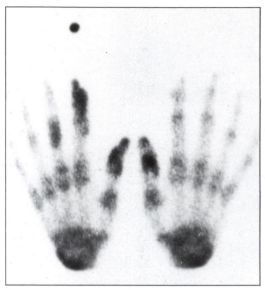

a

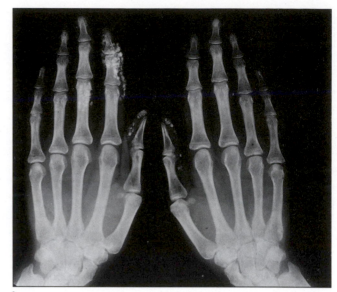

b

**Figure 6.18**

**(a)** Bone scan view of anterior pelvis; **(b)** corresponding X-ray. On the bone scan image a focal area of increased tracer uptake is seen in the right pelvis which is not related to bone. Note also that the bladder is displaced to the left. The X-ray confirms calcification within the right pelvis. The scan and radiographic findings are due to a calcified fibroid. The bladder was being displaced by a large, bulky uterus.

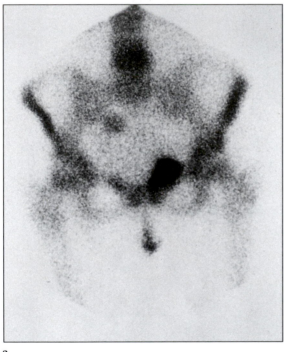

a

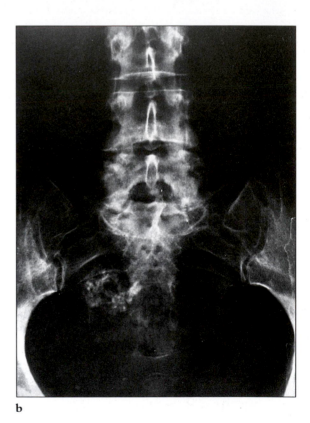

b

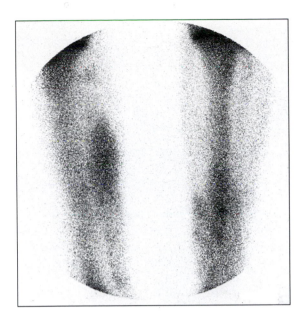

**Figure 6.19**

Soft tissue necrosis. A 16–year-old man who stepped across two adjacent high voltage electrical lines, sustaining deep soft tissue electrical burns in both calves. The $^{99m}$Tc-PYP scan shows soft tissue uptake in both calves, which is more marked on the right.

# ■ Teaching point

■ $^{99m}$Tc-PYP rather than $^{99m}$Tc-MDP is the agent of choice for evaluating soft tissue necrosis. This study may be of value in assessing the extent of soft tissue injury caused by electrical burns. Patients with extensive muscle necrosis may develop renal failure due to myoglobinuria.

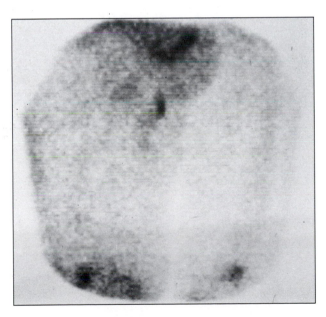

**Figure 6.20**

Lymphoedema. Bone scan view of the femora. It is apparent that there is a marked increase in soft tissue tracer uptake in the right thigh, which in this case was due to lymphoedema.

# Localization of lesion

**Figure 6.21**

An elderly man with known carcinoma of the prostate. Bone scan views: **(a)** skull and anterior cervical spine and **(b)** posterior cervical and thoracic spine. On the anterior view, the appearance might suggest avid tracer accumulation in the thyroid. However, on the posterior view, it is apparent that the lesion lies posteriorly and represents a metastasis in the thoracic spine.

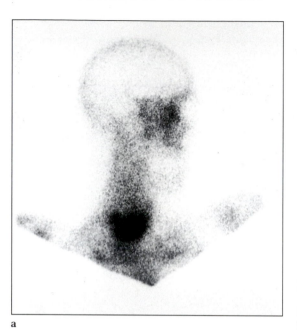

a

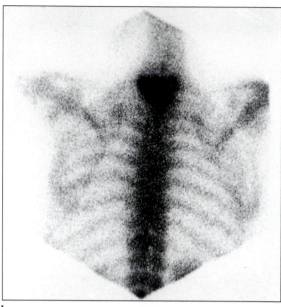

b

# ■ Teaching point

■
Lesions should be visualized in two views whenever possible.

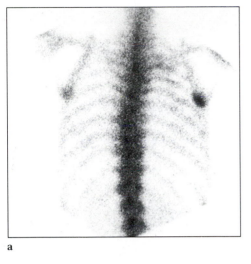

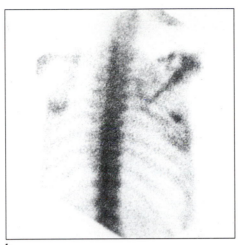

a
b

**Figure 6.22**

Lesion of scapula or rib? Bone scan views: **(a)** thoracic spine and **(b)** with arm elevated. On the original study the lesion appears to lie at the tip of the scapula. However, with the arm elevated, it is apparent that the lesion is in a rib.

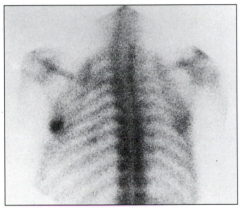

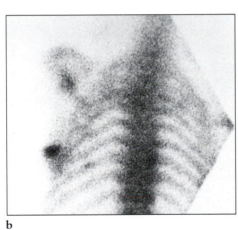

a
b

**Figure 6.23**

Lesion of scapula or rib? Bone scan views: **(a)** posterior thorax and **(b)** with arm elevated. A lesion is seen in the left chest on **(a)** but it is not clear whether it is associated with a rib or the scapula. With the arm elevated, it is apparent that the lesion is in the scapula.

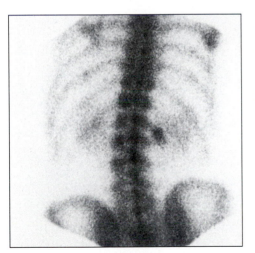

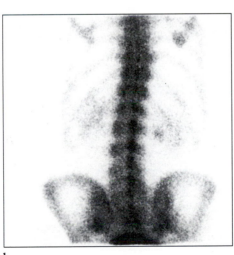

a
b

**Figure 6.24**

Apparent bone lesion accounted for by renal uptake of tracer. Bone scan views: **(a)** supine and **(b)** erect. There is a focal area of increased tracer uptake which appears to overlie the right 12th rib posteriorly. However, this moves with position, and it is clear that the lesion was due to pooling of tracer in the renal pelvis.

# ■ Teaching point

■
On occasion, the precise localization of an abnormality may not be apparent, but will often be clarified if additional views are obtained.

**Figure 6.25**

A 50-year-old man who underwent bone scanning to evaluate the extent of direct invasion by a lacrimal gland adenocystic carcinoma. The tumour, which was causing compression of the posterior and lateral aspect of the left globe, is well shown with magnetic resonance imaging (**a**). Anterior (**b**) and left lateral (**c**) bone scans of the skull were of value in defining the extent of bony involvement prior to surgery.

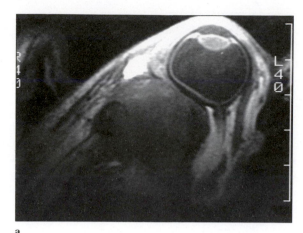

a

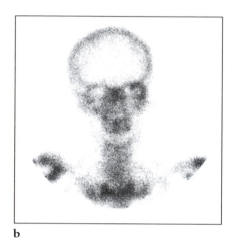

b

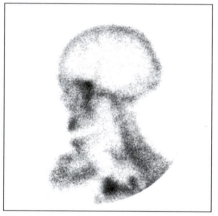

c

# Thoracoplasty

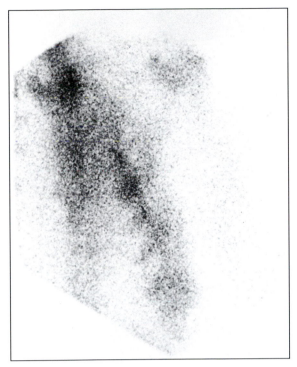

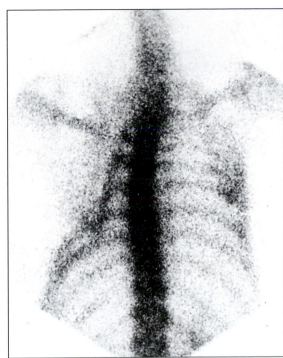

a

b

**Figure 6.26**

Bone scan views: **(a)** left anterior chest and **(b)** posterior thoracic spine. Typical scan appearances of previous thoracoplasty are seen in the left upper ribs.

# Rib resection

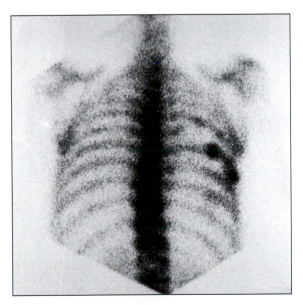

**Figure 6.27**

Bone scan of a patient who had rib resection for plasmacytoma. Note the absence of the right 6th rib posteriorly. Focal abnormalities are seen in the right 5th and 7th ribs posteriorly. There are metabolically active lesions of ribs which are most likely to represent fractures following surgery.

# Vascular abnormalities

**Figure 6.28**

A 54-year-old man who presented 2 years after right total hip replacement complaining of pain in the region of the right groin and greater trochanter. Bone scan views of anterior pelvis and upper femora: **(a)** dynamic and **(b)** delayed. On the dynamic study, the right common iliac artery is not visualized, but there appears to be symmetrical perfusion in the femoral arteries. On static imaging, the appearance of the right prosthesis is unremarkable with no evidence of infection or loosening. An arterial block was subsequently confirmed and the patient's symptoms were attributed to claudication.

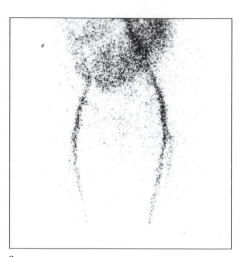

a

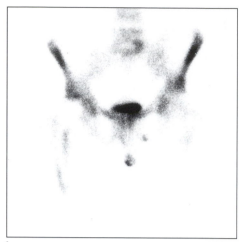

b

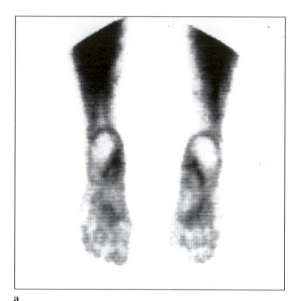

a

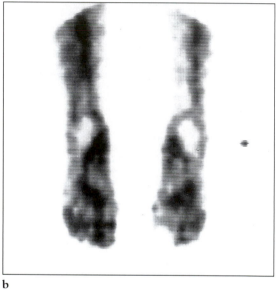

b

**Figure 6.29**

A 22-year-old woman with systemic lupus erythematosus and vasculitis. Bone scan views of feet: **(a)** dynamic, **(b)** blood pool and **(c)** delayed. On the dynamic and blood pool images there is reduced flow to the right 1st and 2nd toes but, on the delayed image, tracer uptake is seen at these sites. However, there are two focal areas of increased uptake seen on the delayed views in the left 2nd and 3rd metatarsophalangeal joints. In the light of the clinical history, the reduced blood flow almost certainly reflects vasculitis. The significance of more focal areas of increased uptake is uncertain but is likely to represent arthritis/degenerative change in the absence of trauma.

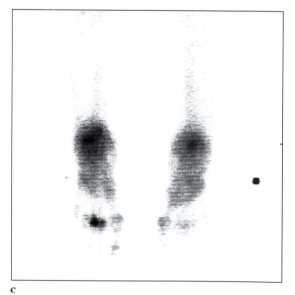

c

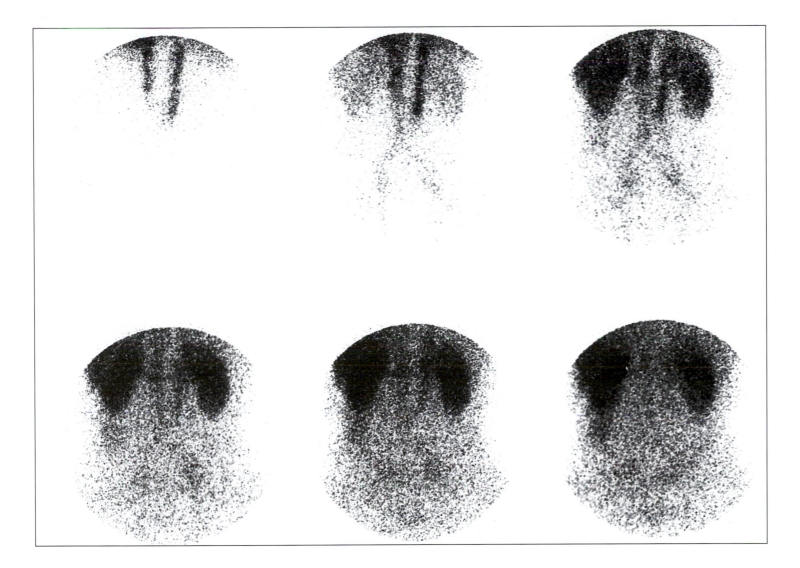

**Figure 6.30**

Visualization of the azygous venous system on the first frame of this dynamic study (5 seconds per frame) of the posterior lumbar spine is a rare but normal finding. This normal variant could be confused with an aorto-caval fistula.

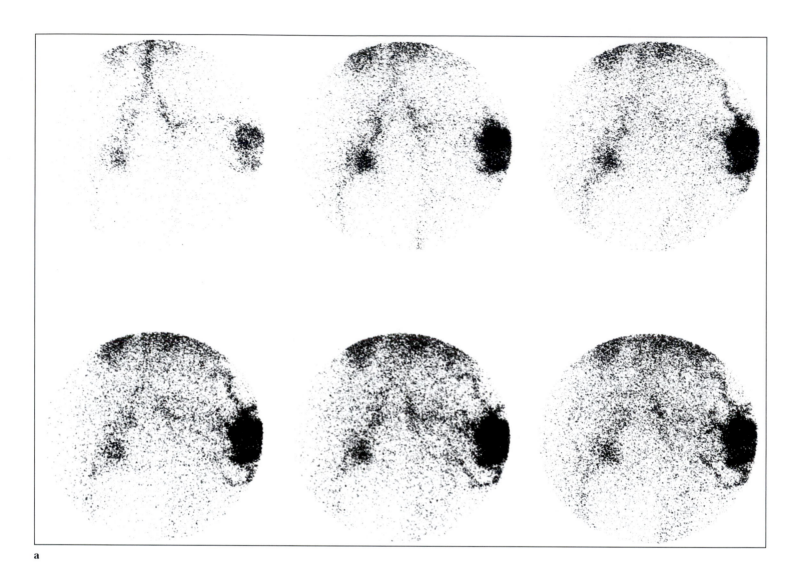

a

## Figure 6.31

Posterior view 5 seconds per frame dynamic study of the pelvis **(a)** in a 72-year-old obese woman shows two highly vascular metastases from renal cell carcinoma. The larger right-sided lesion shows evidence of increased arterial flow, a capillary stain, and early draining veins. Posterior bone scan image **(b)** shows that the left-sided metastasis lies in the left ischium while the right-sided metastasis is in soft tissue. Note the absence of the right kidney.

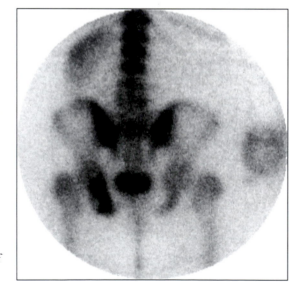

b

# Urinary tract

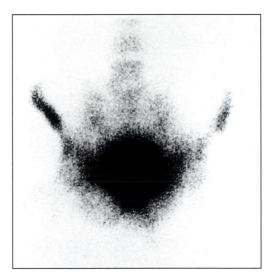

**Figure 6.32**

Full bladder partially obscuring pelvis.

a

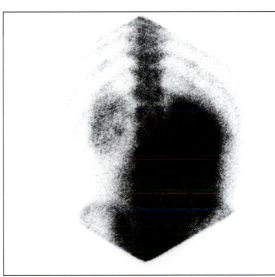

b

**Figure 6.33**

Massive urinary retention. Bone scan views: **(a)** anterior pelvis, **(b)** posterior lumbar spine, and **(c)** right lateral abdomen. The bladder is massively dilated, extending to well above the umbilicus. In addition, there is markedly increased tracer uptake seen in association with the right kidney. The scan findings represent massive urinary retention with some obstruction of the right kidney.

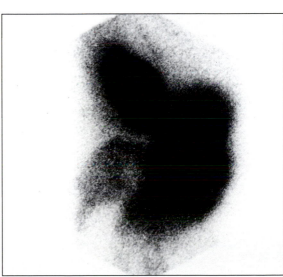

c

**Figure 6.34**

A 76-year-old man with continued left-sided pelvic and hip pain 6 days after a fall. As the patient was unable to adequately empty his bladder, tracer activity within the bladder meant that the pelvis could not be satisfactorily evaluated. A posterior bone scan of the pelvis with a lead shield over the bladder (**a**) shows no abnormality. A 'squat' view of the pelvis could not be obtained due to the patient's pain. However, a posterior bone scan view the next day (**b**) when bladder activity had cleared shows the left-sided pelvic fractures.

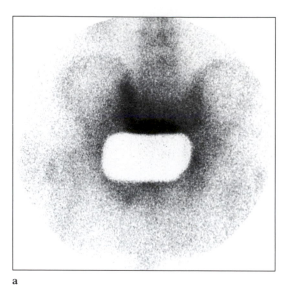

a

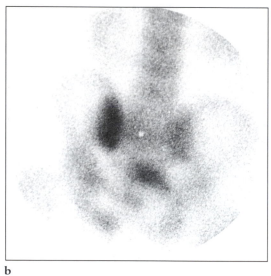

b

# ■ Teaching points

■
Prior to skeletal imaging, a patient should empty the bladder, as retained activity may lead to difficulties in scan interpretation.

■
It is not possible to exclude abnormality in the pelvis unless the bladder is empty. If the bladder obscures the pelvic bones, the patient should be catheterized or a 24-hour delayed view obtained.

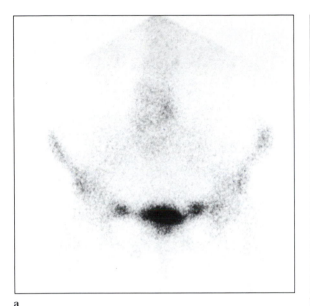

a

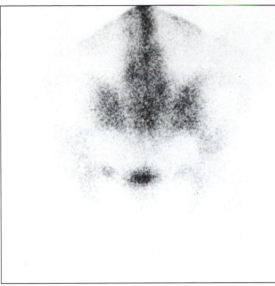

b

**Figure 6.35**

Bladder diverticulae.
Bone scan views:
**(a)** anterior pelvis,
**(b)** posterior pelvis and
**(c)** squat view. On the
anterior and posterior
views of the pelvis, focal
areas of increased tracer
uptake are seen on each
side of the bladder,
overlying the superior
pubic rami. The squat
view clearly separates
these areas from bone and
confirms that these
represent bladder
diverticulae.

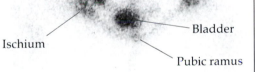

c

**Figure 6.36**

The squat view. A 66-year-old man with a sacral metastasis. Bone scan views: **(a)** anterior, **(b)** posterior and **(c)** squat. There is intensely increased tracer accumulation in the lower sacrum extending throughout the coccyx and the lower portions of both sacroiliac joints. An X-ray confirmed a metastatic deposit at that site. No other lesion was seen throughout the skeleton.

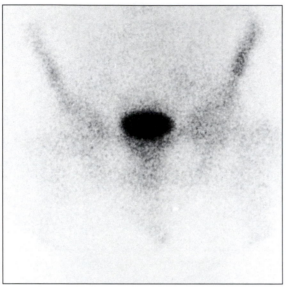

a

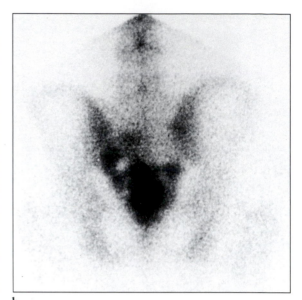

b

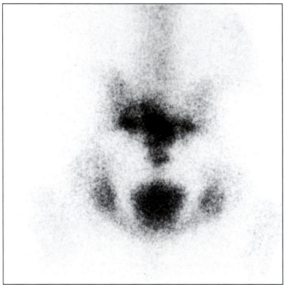

c

## ■ Teaching point

■ Although the scans in Figure 6.36 are obviously abnormal, the study emphasizes the potential importance of obtaining a 'squat' view to separate the bladder from bone. It is possible to imagine a situation where an abnormality is attributed to 'shine through' from the bladder.

# Enlarged prostate

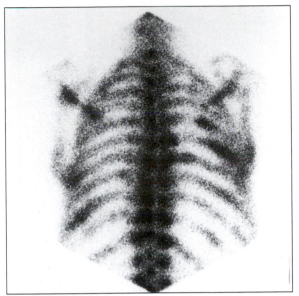

a

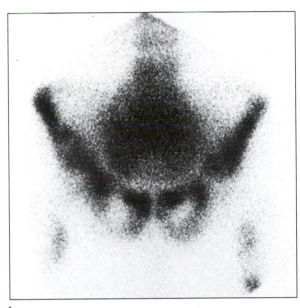

b

**Figure 6.37**

A 75-year-old man with metastatic prostatic carcinoma. Bone scan views: **(a)** posterior thoracic spine and **(b)** anterior pelvis. It is apparent that there is widespread metastatic involvement of the skeleton. In addition, a photon-deficient area is seen at the base of the bladder, which was due to an enlarged prostate. It should be noted that similar, although less prominent, appearances can be found when a patient has an indwelling balloon catheter.

# Metastasis in pubic ramus

**Figure 6.38**

A patient with known carcinoma of the breast. Bone scan views of pelvis: **(a)** anterior, **(b)** posterior and **(c)** squat; **(d)** X-ray of pelvis. The bone scan shows a focal area of increased tracer uptake in the right inferior pubic ramus. In addition, there is increased tracer uptake in the region of the left anterior superior iliac spine. The squat view shows that the lesion overlying the pubic ramus is, indeed, in bone (it is common to see urine contamination). The scan appearances reflect metastatic disease involving the pelvis. The lesion in the right inferior pubic ramus is confirmed on the X-ray.

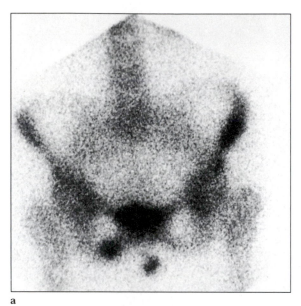

a

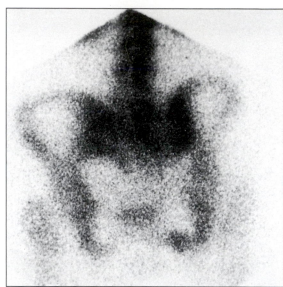

b

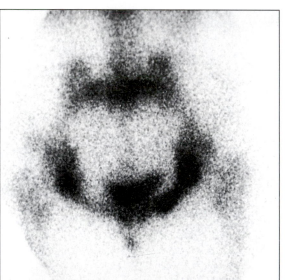

c

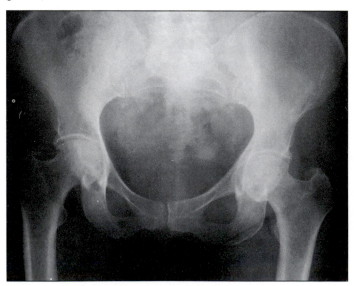

d

# Renal abnormalities

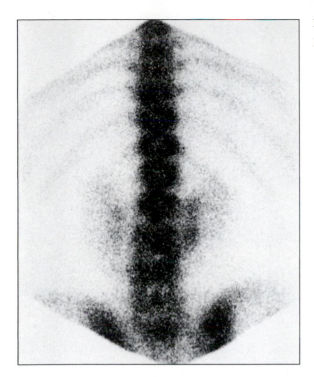

**Figure 6.39**
Horseshoe kidney.

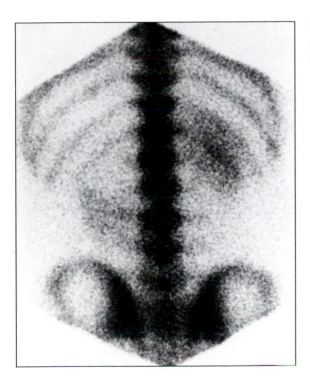

**Figure 6.40**
Hypernephroma of the
left kidney.

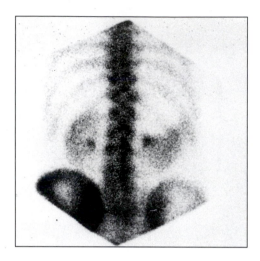

**Figure 6.41**

Cyst in the right kidney

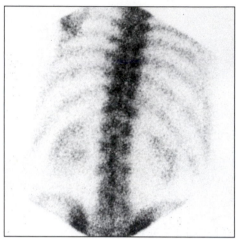

**Figure 6.42**

Renal defect caused by stag-horn calculus.

**Figure 6.43**

Displaced kidney. Bone scan views: **(a)** posterior thoracic/lumbar spine and **(b)** repeat study 4 months later. On the original scan there is a photon-deficient area in T11, and a somewhat less prominent one in T9/T10. Note also that the right kidney is displaced laterally due to a soft tissue mass. This patient had lymphoma, and following radio-therapy lytic disease in the spine persisted, although less prominent than previously. Note also that the right kidney is in a more normal position.

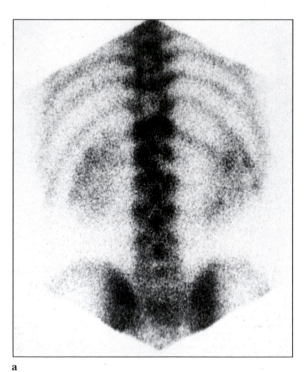

a

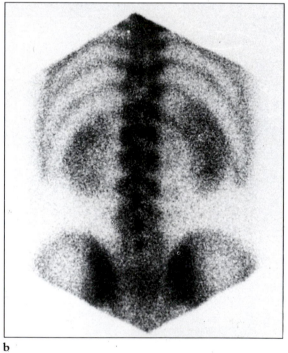

b

# ■ Teaching point

■
Always look at the kidneys.

# Obstructed urinary tract

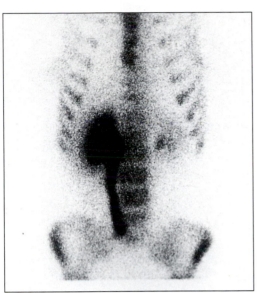

**Figure 6.44**

Anterior bone scan view of lower thorax and abdomen. There is markedly increased tracer uptake in the right kidney and ureter, indicating obstruction at the vesicoureteric junction. This was an incidental finding on an otherwise normal bone scan.

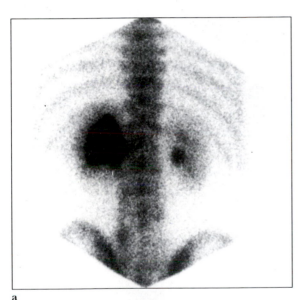

a

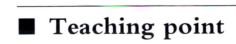

b

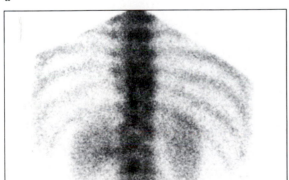

c

**Figure 6.45**

Bone scan views: **(a)** posterior thoracic spine, **(b)** squat view and **(c)** posterior thoracic spine following diuretic. Tracer accumulation is seen in the left renal pelvis, and the lower ureter is prominent. These appearances would be consistent with obstruction at the level of the vesicoureteric junction. However, following diuretic, the tracer is seen to clear. Therefore there is a dilated pelviureteric system which is not obstructed.

## ■ Teaching point

■ The physician should not assume that a dilated collecting system is obstructed.

# Increased renal uptake of diphosphonate caused by hypercalcaemia

**Figure 6.46**

A 67-year-old woman with carcinoma of the breast and hyper-calcaemia. There are multiple focal abnormalities seen throughout the skeleton, attributable to metastases. In addition, there is high uptake of tracer in the kidneys which, in this case, reflects nephrocalcinosis. but may also be found in patients receiving chemotherapy.

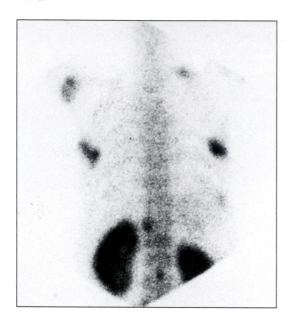

# Urinary diversion

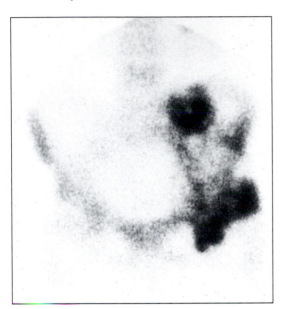

**Figure 6.47**

Anterior bone scan view of pelvis. Tracer uptake is noted in the region of the ileostomy, relating to urinary diversion. Tracer is also seen in the urine bag.

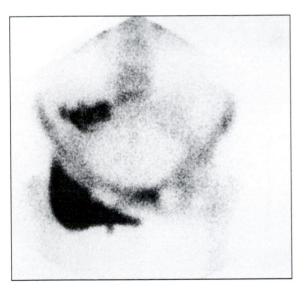

a

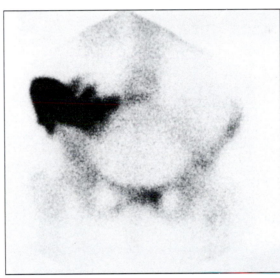

b

**Figure 6.48**

A patient who had urinary diversion carried out for carcinoma of the bladder. **(a)** Anterior bone scan view of the pelvis and **(b)** same view with the urinary collecting bag elevated. In this case, there is a focal lesion in the left pubic ramus caused by a metastasis, and the scan appearances in the left anterior superior iliac spine are also suspicious.

**Figure 6.49**

Caecocystoplasty. Bone scan views: **(a)** anterior and **(b)** posterior pelvis. This patient had a caecocystoplasty performed for carcinoma of the bladder. Marked tracer uptake is seen in the region of the caeococystoplasty, which obscures part of the pelvis.

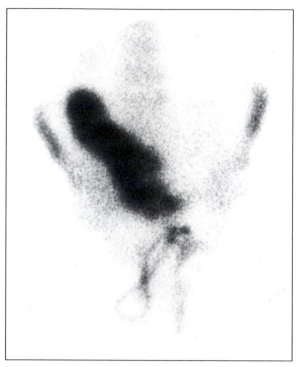

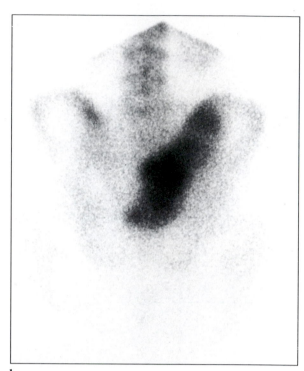

a                                                b

# Acute renal failure

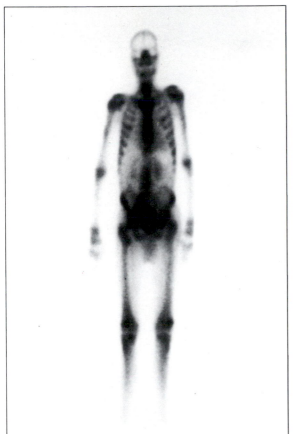

a

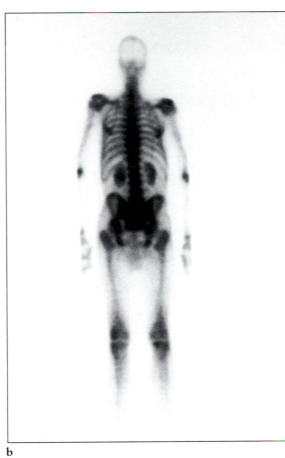

b

**Figure 6.50**

Bone scan views: **(a)** anterior and **(b)** posterior. There is high background tracer activity and the scan appears to be of poor quality. This patient was in acute renal failure at the time of the study.

# Index